MW01143388

HOW DRUGS ARE DEVELOPED

A practical guide to clinical research

David R Hutchinson
BSc PhD MIBiol CBiol FSS

BROOKWOOD MEDICAL PUBLICATIONS

ABOUT THE AUTHOR

D R DAVID HUTCHINSON is an experienced teacher of clinical research. He is an honours graduate in Biochemistry – Toxicology (BSc) and Clinical Biochemistry (PhD) from the University of Surrey, a Fellow of the Royal Statistical Society and a Fellow of the Royal Society of Medicine. After working as a clinical trials organiser and Head of Clinical Research in the pharmaceutical industry and in contract clinical research for more than 12 years, he is now Director of the Brookwood International Academy of Healthcare Research. Dr Hutchinson has presented clinical research topics in the UK, Europe, Scandinavia, South Korea, Japan and the USA. He teaches clinical research and GCP to the pharmaceutical industry, investigators and university students. As well as publishing numerous articles reporting clinical trial results and clinical trial methodology, Dr Hutchinson is author of *A Practical Guide to GCP for Investigators*, *The Trial Investigator's GCP Handbook* and *Which Documents, Why?* and co-author of *Dictionary of Clinical Research*.

ACKNOWLEDGMENTS

I am grateful to Anne Guiry, Neil Mountain and
Ben Saunders for their valuable assistance in the production
of this publication.

I am also grateful to my 'mentor' Dr Paul Marcus without
whom none of my experience would have been gained.

CONTENTS

CHAPTER 1. The fundamentals of clinical research   **1**

INTRODUCTION **1**

DRUG DEVELOPMENT AND THE PHARMACEUTICAL INDUSTRY **1**

Drug discovery 2
Initial tests 2
First administration to Man – Phase I 3
First administration to patients – Phase II 3
Risk-benefit ratio 4
Difficult decisions 5
Larger scale studies of efficacy and safety – Phase III 5
Application for a product licence 5
Post-marketing studies – Phase IV 6
Health economics 7
The need for cost effective research 7

THE ELEMENTS OF CLINICAL RESEARCH **8**

Patient protection in clinical trials 8
Regulatory aspects 9
The clinical trial protocol 10
Case record forms 11
Trial objectives 13
Controls 14
Trial design 15
Multicentre studies 17
Allocating treatment 18
Blinding 20
Obtaining balanced treatment groups 20
Variability in medicine 21
Placebo 22
Placebo response 22
Using placebo in double blind studies 24
Payment in clinical trials 24

MEASUREMENT IN CLINICAL TRIALS **26**

Measuring efficacy 26
Measuring safety 28
Adverse events 29

CHAPTER 2. The critical path of the clinical trial   **32**

INTRODUCTION **32**
STAGES OF THE CLINICAL TRIAL **34**
  Planning 34
  The study protocol 35
  Case record forms 36
  Ethics and regulatory affairs 36
  Selection of investigators 38
  Site assessment and pre-study briefing 39
  Study materials 39
  Patient recruitment 40
  Periodic monitoring 42
  Study termination 43
  Data entry and statistical analysis 43
  The Final Report 44

CHAPTER 3. Good clinical practice   **46**

INTRODUCTION **46**
  The need for good clinical practice 46
  What is good clinical practice? 47
  Harmonisation of GCP? 48
  Standard Operating Procedures 50
  Responsibilities 50

OUTLINE OF ICH GOOD CLINICAL PRACTICE GUIDELINES **51**
  Protection of trial subjects and consultation of Ethics Committees..... 51
  Responsibilities 52
  Data handling 55
  Statistics 56
  Quality assurance 57
  The Trial Master File 58
  Problems of implementing GCP 58
  Conclusion 59

CHAPTER 4. Further reading   **61**

APPENDICES **63**
INDEX **77**

1

The fundamentals of clinical research

INTRODUCTION

Clinical research is part of the complex procedure to demonstrate the effectiveness and safety of drugs and other products of the pharmaceutical industry. It requires the collaboration of many personnel with a variety of skills. A good clinical research team is based on reliability and the non-technical staff have as great a role to play as the medically and scientifically qualified personnel who manage the programme. It is essential, therefore, that the secretaries, administrators and other members of the team are fully aware of the procedures of clinical research and, in particular, the rules placed upon their actions by Good Clinical Practice and Standard Operating Procedures.

DRUG DEVELOPMENT AND THE PHARMACEUTICAL INDUSTRY

It should never be forgotten that the pharmaceutical company, like all other businesses, is a commercial concern and strives to make a profit as a result of its trading. The prime aim of a pharmaceutical company must therefore be to develop or buy-in and then sell products at a profit. With this in mind, the search for new drugs and their successful development is a future source of income for the company. Of, perhaps, 10,000 molecules which are screened as potential new products, laboratory tests then identify a few compounds, maybe 15 or so, that seem worthy of further study.

After early evaluations in animals a few of these will eventually be given to Man, leading to one or two new products for future development. The cost of the search for these compounds is likely to be in the order of several billion pounds. Careful planning of resources and clinical research programmes is important to minimise the research and development costs, without risk to the patient, so as to maximise the profits as a result of future sales.

Most drugs sold by the pharmaceutical company have been developed by the research teams of that company. Not all drugs are found by this route, however. Alternatively, the company may sell *generics,* ie. drugs that have been developed by another company but whose patent has expired, allowing other companies to manufacture and market the same drug but at a much cheaper price. Drugs may also be "licensed-in": this involves an agreement between two pharmaceutical companies whereby one company allows the other to manufacture and sell a product "owned" by the former company.

In this book we will only consider the development of a drug from the company's own research and development activities.

Drug discovery

Studies of the actions of synthetically made chemical structures can be used to predict the molecules likely to have a therapeutic effect, ie. have a beneficial effect in Man. Computers may be used to design the chemical structures of new molecules and predict their therapeutic activities and side effect profiles; these can then be made in small quantities in the laboratory. Hundreds of new compounds are produced in the search for a single active substance.

Initial tests

Most new molecules are administered to specially bred animals in carefully controlled environments. These tests are important to discover which drugs are likely to be the most effective and safe when given to Man. Although the use of animals in laboratory experiments is controversial and generally undesirable, there is currently no other system that allows the evaluation of new drugs with the same degree of reliability or acceptability to government Boards of Health.

Studies are undertaken on a new compound to determine how much can be administered without side effects occurring, to determine whether or not the new compound causes cancer or other serious toxicity and to determine the effect of the substance on reproduction (teratology). In recent times these tests have become more rigorous in an attempt to prevent the latter horrors of side effects caused by drugs such as thalidomide and more recently benoxaprofen. On the basis of animal tests, compounds are selected for further study in Man.

First administration to Man – Phase I

Small amounts of drug are administered in controlled circumstances to a few carefully selected and screened healthy volunteers. Blood levels of drug, the excretion characteristics and any beneficial or unwanted effects are monitored in order to evaluate the behaviour of the drug in Man. As confidence about the safety of the new drug grows, higher doses are used and multiple doses are administered to the volunteers. Some idea about the minimum and maximum doses of drug is obtained to identify an optimum dose to use in further research in patients.

This first administration in Man is termed *"Phase I"* in the drug development pathway.

First administration to patients – Phase II

The use of healthy volunteers provides information about the dose of drug required to give reasonable blood levels, ie.

pharmacokinetic data. It is usually impossible to demonstrate a therapeutic action in healthy individuals. The second stage of drug development, *"Phase II"*, involves giving the drug to a small number of patient volunteers. The pharmacokinetics and excretion of the drug are re-evaluated, because drugs are often handled differently by the body when an illness is present, especially those affecting the stomach, intestines, liver or kidney.

Consider, for example, the development of a new pain-killer, an analgesic, for the treatment of arthritis. The Phase II studies will determine how effective the new drug is at relieving pain in patients with arthritis. These studies will also demonstrate the incidence of side effects at different doses and help to establish the *"optimum dose"* at which pain is adequately relieved with the minimum number of side effects.

Risk-benefit ratio

The benefits obtained by taking a drug for the treatment of a certain condition should always outweigh the risk of taking that drug. Take for example a simple pain relieving drug; if you took this drug for the treatment of a headache it would be quite unacceptable if a side effect of treatment was massive hair loss. On the other hand, a patient with terminal cancer would almost certainly accept terrible side effects of treatment in return for a total cure of their condition. These examples demonstrate that each drug and therapeutic area has different acceptable risk-benefits; in the development of a new drug, consideration will always be given to the risks and benefits of alternative treatments (including similar drugs already available for use) before deciding whether or not to proceed with further development. A drug with an unacceptable risk-benefit ratio will not be approved by regulatory authorities and in any case it is unlikely to be used by the medical profession if better products are available.

Difficult decisions

After the first two phases of drug development the company must decide whether or not to proceed with further development of the product. Millions of pounds have already been spent by this time and if the decision is not to proceed it is very painful financially. The reasons for discontinuation with the project would include: poor tolerability leading to high number of side effects; formulation of the drug not stable or palatable; little or no effectiveness; cost of production outweighing the projected income; the drug being inferior to similar compounds.

If the drug appears worthy of further development, more clinical studies are undertaken in order to prove its effectiveness, ie. its efficacy, and its safety (tolerability) in larger numbers of patients.

Larger scale studies of efficacy and safety – Phase III

These studies are undertaken in hospital and general practice to confirm the efficacy and tolerability of a drug in large numbers of patients. Clinical trials to compare these parameters with placebo – an inactive substance – and with similar drugs already on the market are performed. The results should be reproducible from study to study. This is the busiest and most intensive part of a clinical research programme. In addition to studies on adult sick patients, special studies to check the safety of the drug in elderly patients and sometimes in children are also undertaken. On the whole, elderly and severely sick patients require smaller doses of drug as their bodies are unable to clear drugs effectively; this may mean that elderly patients are more likely to suffer from side effects and special investigations are therefore justified.

Application for a product licence

The data on many thousands of treated subjects are evaluated in

Phases I to III and reports prepared. These, together with all the data from animal and laboratory studies (ie. pre-clinical data), are sent, in the UK, to the Department of Health, Medicines Control Agency (MCA) for evaluation by a team of experts. Usually this evaluation takes many months, or even years, and if the drug is considered to be effective, safe and useful a Product Licence (PL) will be granted which allows the company to sell the drug, usually on a prescription only basis, and only for the treatment of the conditions which have been studied in clinical trials. Drugs for the treatment of AIDS and cancer are considered more quickly than those in some other therapeutic areas where adequate treatments are currently available.

Post-marketing studies – Phase IV

Once a company has a PL further research is still required. Some of this is termed *"Phase IV"* research. Phase IV studies are usually undertaken in close collaboration with the marketing department, whose main interest is in the growth of product sales; Phase IV studies are often thought of as "marketing studies" and compare a product with its competitors. The previously undertaken clinical trials will have evaluated the drug in special groups of patients, carefully selected, with many exclusions. Once available on prescription, many different types of patient will receive the drug. It is important, therefore, to evaluate further the efficacy and tolerability of the new drug in larger numbers of people. Companies often set up "Post-Marketing Surveillance Studies" (PMS) in order to do this. In these studies data on many thousands of patients treated with the drug are collected and analysed. Previously undetected side effects with a low incidence may be observed. These data will support those already collected in clinical trials and will enable the company to make prescribers aware of the risks and benefits of treatment in the "normal patient population" more reliably.

Another reason for performing further studies is to extend the range of indications for which the drug may be used. The PL clearly defines the illnesses which may be treated with the drug; many other indications may also be treated but the evidence of clinical trials is required first. Take our previous example of the new analgesic for the treatment of arthritis; we may now undertake trials in sports injuries, back pain, and general aches and pains in order to extend the useful range of indications the drug may be used to treat. If these studies show that the drug is effective in the treatment of these conditions, an extension to the PL may be applied for. Studies such as these widen the application of the drug and therefore increase the potential market and future sales. In some companies, these studies on new indications are classed as *"Phase IV"* whilst others class them *"Phase IIIB"* (*"Phase IIIA"* being the earlier studies on other indications).

Health economics

An increasing trend in clinical research is to demonstrate that a new product is cost effective to use. Government pressures on prescribing doctors to use the cheapest available option (providing the drugs compared have similar efficacy/safety) have led pharmaceutical companies to perform economic exercises to show that by using their new product a doctor can save money. Some important justifications to offset the high cost of new drugs include the cost of treating side effects, shorter hospital stays and less recurrence of the treated condition. In some countries (eg. Canada, Australia) companies are compelled to undertake health economic evaluations in order to justify their product licence application.

The need for cost effective research

In the past, clinical trials have been undertaken because "it would be nice to know what happens". With increasing costs in the development of a new drug, the luxury of performing trials for this reason has gone. Carefully planned clinical trial programmes must ensure that the drug reaches the market in as short a time as possible. Well designed trials with clear objectives, and consultation with the marketing department in order to work towards a common goal, are essential.

The selection of therapeutic area is vastly dependent on the overall size of the market, the share expected and the cost of development. Little research will be undertaken on drugs competing in a generic market (eg. benzodiazepine hypnotics) where the cost of competitive products is low and, therefore, does not allow a company to recoup the research costs and make a profit.

Inevitably the number of clinical trials in commonly researched areas is great and competition between companies for investigators and patients is fierce. This leads to high fees being paid to investigators and potentially unethical payments being made in order that one trial is undertaken in preference to another.

Although the need for clinical trials to show efficacy and safety is great, the temptation to perform badly designed, unethical studies must be avoided. The costs of wasted and badly performed research can no longer be a part of the modern research and development programme. It is the duty of all staff involved in clinical research, therefore, to ensure that resources are not wasted, deadlines and objectives are met and clinical trials are conducted to the highest standards.

THE ELEMENTS OF CLINICAL RESEARCH

Patient protection in clinical trials

Clinical trials are the only means by which the efficacy and safety of drugs are investigated in Man. They inevitably carry risk to those who take part, to the investigator and to the company which sponsors the study. The risk to the volunteer or patient should be minimised by careful selection of those who are treated, but compensation should be available to those who suffer adverse events during a clinical trial. The risk to the investigator should be covered by the sponsor accepting strict liability for any untoward events occurring during the study, and the risk to the sponsor should be carefully calculated by the company before embarking on any project.

All patients who are considered for recruitment to a clinical trial must be asked for their consent before any trial procedures are undertaken. This process is called *"obtaining informed consent"*. The study protocol must also be reviewed by an independent panel called an Ethics Committee: medical professionals and lay people, of both sexes and a suitable representation of different ages and races, should make up this committee, which is often formed and controlled by an Area or Regional Health Authority. The Ethics Committee will decide whether or not the study should be allowed to be performed, and will seek to ensure the maximum protection of those who take part in the study. Patients are also protected by the Declaration of Helsinki. These elements are discussed in more detail later in this book.

Regulatory aspects

Before a study of an unlicensed drug can start in patients (ie. Phases II and III), the approval of the Board of Health must be obtained. In the UK the Department of Health Medicines, Control Agency (MCA) has this role; in the USA the Food and Drugs Administration (FDA) has a similar function.

The Clinical Trial Exemption (CTX) Scheme is now the most common method of obtaining approval in the UK. The trial sponsor submits a package of summarised data together with names of investigators and the protocol for the study it wishes to undertake. Approval is usually granted within 35 days unless further time for consideration is requested. This approval allows the company to recruit and treat only the patients specified in the protocol and each study must be submitted in this way.

In the USA, the trial sponsor makes an IND (Investigational New Drug) application.

Legislation through a European Directive (1997) is likely to require Phase I studies to be approved by the regulatory authorities. Prior to this, approval of Phase I studies was not required in the UK.

The clinical trial protocol

The key to a successful clinical trial is a realistic well written protocol. Often a company has an "in house" style but the contents of the protocol will be similar from company to company and centre to centre. A Standard Operating Procedure, explained later, should be in force determining how a protocol should be written and prepared. You should make yourself aware of these "rules" as detailed advice will be given about style, format and section headings.

Some general tips on protocol preparation include the following:

● try to avoid repetition
● a good structure and clear headings will assist the investigator
● protocol summaries may be provided and a "flowchart" to show the times of important assessments is helpful
● remember to append essential documents, eg. Declaration of Helsinki, ABPI Codes of Practice, ABPI Guidelines on Liability; these are often forgotten.

While the protocol is being prepared, you should avoid the temptation to "cannibalise" another previously prepared one which may be similar. This may give rise to major errors which can be included, never detected and subsequently undertaken in the study (and in future studies!). Every statement in the protocol should be thought about to ensure that it is appropriate. For example, all too common is the use of exclusion criteria from protocol to protocol, passed on without any thought as to the applicability to the study. The ultimate cost is that patients are erroneously excluded from the study, thus reducing the available patient population and extending the time needed to recruit patients. Remember, lost time is lost income from sales. Standard blocks of text regarding administration of the study, adverse event reporting and so on may be set up as macros on a computer and used from protocol to protocol, providing the author checks the relevance of these statements.

The protocol is the "recipe" or working document that all investigators agree to adhere to when performing a clinical trial. It is important that the protocol is read and understood by the investigator. The best protocols usually have some investigator input, helping to make them practical and manageable. Presentation of the document is extremely important – try to use a readable font style and size; personally I find single spaced Courier difficult to read and prefer Times. The use of clear headings and short paragraphs will help the reader.

Case record forms

The design of record books (usually called case record forms, case report forms or CRFs) is another matter for which teamwork is important. The record card or booklet should lend itself to ease of coding and transition between the paper based system and the computer. The statistician should be part of the design team.

The use of self-duplicating (NCR) paper in CRFs is common. There are many pitfalls in its use but it provides multiple copies of the data collected in a trial, which is often a useful safeguard. After each patient is entered, or at the end of the trial, a copy can be sent to the company whilst the investigator keeps a copy for himself. Beware though – NCR paper may fade with time, like fax paper, and so second and third copies may end up blank. There is one rule which must never, ever be broken: do not allow the only copy of the data to be sent in the post or by courier, particularly if this is done in a batch, just in case the data gets lost.

A good deal of thought must go into the design of the CRF book in terms of its simplicity and acceptability by the person whose job it is to fill it in – the investigator. The busy clinician will be more likely to generate 'clean' data if the record book makes this easy for him/her, and there are many ways in which this can be achieved, for instance:

- printing the units of measurements so that they do not have to be written
- including a flowchart which shows the order in which measurements must be taken
- allowing adequate space for data to be collected
- producing simple and easy to follow forms, not too busy or "frightening".

Each point may be trivial in itself, but together they make a large difference to the success of the study. The temptation is to collect more clinical data than are absolutely necessary. Richard Peto has rightly said, "The statistician should, at the design stage, cross out from the draft coding forms most of the things that the trial organiser thinks he wants to ask".

The design of the record form may be one of the most potent factors in deciding whether a consultant agrees to participate in a trial. If possible, the layout and presentation of the form should be visually attractive and the form of printing and duplication chosen suitable for the purpose intended. For instance, a large multicentre general practice study would demand very different record forms compared with a smaller trial carried out in a specialist hospital unit. Above all, the record forms should not be ambiguous. Only the information which is absolutely necessary should be requested and it should be perfectly clear where this should be entered and in what units it should be expressed.

Some thought should be given to where to place boxes to record data on a page, what shape and how large to make them, how many lines to leave, the space between lines, the position of alternatives to tick or cross, and so on. The good use of fonts, boldface and italics may enhance instructions or other text. The precision with which data are recorded should not be left to the discretion of the form-filler. Thus, whether the investigator is to round to whole numbers or use decimal places or fractions must be specified, or else doubts will be raised in the investigator's mind and there will be considerable difficulty when the data come to be processed. Great care must be taken with linguistics so that the meaning of instructions is absolutely clear. This is particularly the case in any sort of documentation intended for use by patients whose intellect and scientific background may be very different from that of the person compiling the record form. It is essential that each page of the CRF is uniquely identified – the patient's initials, date of visit, study code, centre number and page number should be included.

The ultimate test of the suitability of the CRF is to complete it yourself and ask others to do the same – it will amaze you!

Overall, the success of a trial depends on the design of the CRF. A poorly designed form will not be completed reliably, leading to poor data collection and a likely erroneous trial result. Care and attention in the presentation of the CRF is vital to the success of the study.

Trial objectives

It cannot be emphasised enough that each trial should have a clear aim or objective. The study is likely to address some of the following questions (not every one in each study):

- Is the treatment of therapeutic value? Does it work?
- How does it compare with other products or placebo?
- Which type of patients benefit most?
- What is the optimum dose and route of administration?
- What is the safety profile of the drug and what are the key adverse drug reactions?

"A formal trial should have a precisely framed question and have equivalent groups treated concurrently but different treatments with random allocation" (Bradford Hill).

Once it has been decided that a clinical trial must be carried out to answer some valid therapeutic question, the form that the trial will take must be planned. There are a large number of ways of setting up a clinical investigation, and some of the concepts will be dealt with here.

Controls

A control substance should always be given to patients within a study for comparative purposes with the treatment under investigation. Controls may be 'active' – often the most commonly used drug for the particular condition under study or the market leader/standard – or 'inactive' (placebo). Particularly in the early stages of drug development, trials with inactive controls are preferred to demonstrate that drug activity is greater than that explained by placebo response. In the later phases of research, active controls are more often used, because they give information which will be of value in marketing. It is essential to ensure that the comparisons are relevant: that the correct drug and the correct dosage are used. Choosing correct dosages of new drugs under study and the right comparative dose of active control is often difficult early on, when pharmacological and pharmacodynamic data may be available from volunteers but the correct dose in patients may not be known. In this situation it is best to do a smaller dose finding study first, or the comparison may be unfair.

It is common for all patients who are recruited to a study to first of all enter a *"run-in"* phase of treatment during which placebo or no treatment is taken. This eliminates the effects of any previous treatments that may have been taken and provides an opportunity to undertake baseline reference measures of the patients condition before taking the trial drugs.

Trial design

When comparing two different drug treatments, patients may be given only one of the drugs or alternatively given both treatments on different occasions. Groups of patients are used and the two techniques are known as *"parallel group"* or *"crossover"* designs.

● *Crossover studies*

In the crossover study of two drugs (A and B), each patient takes both drugs, one after the other (Figures 1 and 2). The order in which the treatments are given is randomly decided (to avoid the best or worse drug always being taken first, thereby eliminating any bias in the results obtained from the alternative treatment). The crossover study has a number of advantages and also some disadvantages in comparison with the parallel group design. Although there may be a saving in terms of the number of patients required for the trial, the greatest concern is that the baseline state at the beginning of the second treatment period may not be the same as that at the start of the first. As Confucius said: "You cannot dip your finger in the same river twice". The disease itself may have changed during the first treatment period, or there may be a carry-over effect of one treatment after the next has been instituted. Because of this, it may be necessary to have a *"wash-out"* period between the two treatments (ie. a period of taking

FIGURE 1. Crossover study with no run-in and no wash-out.

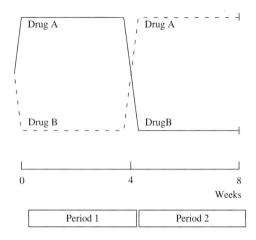

FIGURE 2. Crossover study with run-in and wash-out.

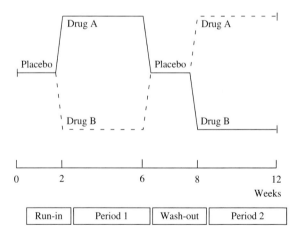

placebo, no medication or a mild, non-competing drug which satisfies the needs of the patient in minimising discomfort), as it may have been before the first was given. This may not, however, be feasible.

Another concern, in the longer trial, is the effect of seasonal variation on the patient's condition. In general, crossover studies (also called within-patient comparisons) should be as short as possible, but even so this method of trial design is becoming less favoured.

The best use of the crossover design is in the palliative treatment of chronic diseases.

● *Parallel group design*
In a parallel group study of two drugs (A and B) each patient takes only one of the study medications (either A or B). An example of a parallel group design in shown in Figure 3. In this design one group of patients receives one treatment and another group receives the alternative medication. This is the most commonly used trial design. Here the danger is of having an imbalance of relevant factors in the two groups and special kinds of parallel group design are occasionally used.

The *"matched pair"* study has been developed as a way of trying to overcome this problem. Here pairs of patients are selected, chosen for their similarity in key factors such as age, sex, duration and severity of disease, and so on. These are then randomly allocated to treatment with either drug. The disadvantage of this technique is the delay involved in finding matches for specific patients. An extreme example of the technique is to recruit identical twins. If these studies can practically be set up they are often very successful. Matched pair studies are rarely used for practical reasons.

Multicentre studies

All the above designs may be used on a single or multicentre basis. Multicentre trials are more difficult to carry out than those at a single establishment. It is often extremely difficult to agree the protocol, and the administrative, logistical and communication problems are severe. At least some aspects of the study which are common to all

FIGURE 3. Parallel group study with run-in.

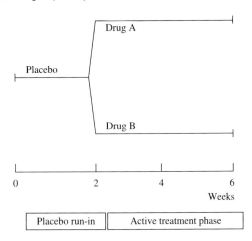

centres *must* be agreed – "core criteria". In a formal multicentre trial investigators should ideally meet and agree the protocol, and this should be followed by regular discussions between investigators, statisticians and trial monitors as the study progresses.

Allocating treatment

In normal medical practice, it is the prescriber who decides which drug each particular patient will receive. In controlled trials, the only decision the prescriber makes is whether or not a particular patient satisfies the inclusion criteria for the trial. Thereafter the drug he/she receives, or the one he/she receives first, is decided on the basis of a list of treatments, usually in random order. The allocation of treatments must be by chance, and there are a number of ways of achieving this: spinning a coin, consulting tables of random numbers, using a computer, drawing papers out of a hat, etc.

Usually these randomisation schedules are prepared in 'blocks' of patients. In a 'block' of six patients, for example, three would receive treatment A and three would receive treatment B. Treatments are randomised within each block. Blocks are used to ensure that, as a study progresses, approximately equal numbers of patients have received each treatment.

It is important that treatments are allocated in strict numerical order otherwise imbalance in the number of patients receiving each treatment may occur.

Where there is likely to be a difference in response between sub-groups of patients within the same group it is necessary to stratify the randomisation list. For example, if males and females are likely to respond in different ways it is necessary to have a random list for male patients and female patients in each group to avoid imbalance which would be caused by, for example, all male patients taking treatment A and all females taking treatment B (see Figure 4).

FIGURE 4. A stratified random code in blocks of six patients.

MALES		FEMALES	
Patient number	**Treatment**	**Patient number**	**Treatment**
1m	A	1f	B
2m	A	2f	A
3m	B	3f	B
4m	A	4f	A
5m	B	5f	A
6m	B	6f	B

Male patients are allocated numbers 1m to 6m, females are allocated patient numbers 1f to 6f. Within each strata therefore, equal numbers of males and females will receive each treatment.

Blinding

Usually the investigator is *"blind"*, such that he/she does not see the list which is held by a dispenser. In the *"double blind"* study neither the patient nor the investigator (and preferably the study monitor and other company personnel involved in the day-to-day management of the study) know which treatment is being taken. The purpose of this is to avoid bias on the part of patient or doctor in assessing the results of treatment. Elaborate precautions are often required to preserve blinding, such as formulating the drug and the control substance (active or inactive) in an identical way so that they look, feel and taste the same.

It is important for provision to be made so that the code can be broken for an individual patient in the case of an emergency. Usually each patient's treatment is marked on a piece of paper in an individual sealed envelope. These "patient codes" should be tamper-proof in opaque "lick" sealed envelopes – some investigators and monitors like to break the code as the study progresses and this is strictly not allowed.

In an *"open"* study the investigator and patient are aware what medication is being taken. These studies are least reliable as bias may affect the outcome.

A halfway house is the *"single blind"* study when the patient or assessor (preferably) is unaware of the medication being taken. Although this goes some way to minimising bias it is not foolproof and the best, most respected studies are undertaken in double blind fashion.

Obtaining balanced treatment groups

Randomisations are usually balanced to ensure that, overall, the same number of patients receive one treatment as receive the other.

The dispensing list as generated above is simple or "non-stratified". A "stratified" randomisation can be utilised to minimise the risk of imbalance or bias occurring because of the preponderance of a particular factor relevant to the disease or its treatment in one or other treatment group. To do this, patients are first of all separated into groups according to the factors which are important (examples would be male and female, above and below 65 years of age, duration of illness greater or less than six months), and then each group of patients has its own randomisation list prepared for it.

Statisticians refer to the number of levels within a stratification (eg. sex has two levels – male and female). Permutation of the levels arising from different relevant factors gives rise to "sub-groups". The number of sub-groups increases, obviously, as the number of factors taken into account increases, and very complex patterns may quickly be reached, with practical difficulties in administration and statistical ones in analysis. A reasonable compromise needs to be agreed between the clinician, the monitor and the statistician. In multicentre trials each centre should be regarded as different, and a whole block of randomisation should be given to it, with the appropriate stratification as required included.

Variability in medicine

If a bar of a certain metal is heated through a certain temperature rise time and time again, it will always expand by precisely the same amount. If other bars of the same material are heated to the same temperature, the same expansion will be measured. Experimentation in physics and chemistry may be said to be relatively simple because the effects are strictly reproducible.

This is not the case in biology and in medicine in particular. Different patients with the same disease will behave differently in response to drug treatment, and the same patient may behave differently on different occasions. It has been said that *"There is no always or never in medicine"*. This is one of the main reasons for the need for formal therapeutic trials, and for the requirement to include large groups of patients treated under double blind controlled conditions.

Placebo

Active drugs are often compared with placebo. This is made to resemble the active substance, but is without therapeutic effect and is needed because it is known that even an inactive substance may produce considerable benefit when given to a patient, especially if it is accompanied by an optimistic manner on the part of the prescriber. The word placebo comes from the Latin *"placere"* which means "to please". Placebos are widely used therapeutically, sometimes intentionally but more often in the expectation that the substance concerned is active in a particular patient when in fact it is not; an example would be tonics. Use of the placebo response may represent between 20 and 40% of all prescriptions. Placebo preparations may take any formulation (tablet, capsule, injection, elixir).

Placebo response

Placebo response arises from the patient's belief or faith in a medicine, and is now thought to be caused by the release of active endorphins in various parts of the brain. The action of the placebo substance can be enhanced by "the power of positive prescribing": the confident manner of the physician suggesting that he definitely expects benefits to accrue. Placebo substances can have a variety of subjective effects, as has been demonstrated by a number of careful clinical trials:

- one-third of asthmatic attacks have been relieved by saline injection in one study
- placebo as well as codeine has been shown to suppress coughing

- headache may respond to placebo in as many as 50% of cases
- post-operative pain showed a 15 – 20% placebo response.

Even objective effects may be recorded:

- placebo may lower blood pressure in patients with essential hypertension
- a placebo injection has improved exercise tolerance in a physiological experiment
- an endoscopic study of the gastric mucosa has shown clear effects from placebo
- a rise in circulating eosinophils was found with placebo in a study on schizophrenia
- in a study of the hormone ACTH on adrenocortical function in anxious patients, placebo brought about an increase in neutrophils and a decrease in lymphocytes and eosinophils.

Placebo can cause a wide range of side effects in clinical trials, including:

- depression of the CNS (drowsiness, fatigue, unsteady gait, motor retardation)
- stimulation of the CNS, including nervousness, excitement and motor agitation
- gastrointestinal side effects (nausea, anorexia, constipation)
- dry mouth.

It should be noted that colour, shape, taste and formulation can greatly influence placebo response.

The setting (on the ward, in the home or at work) will also influence placebo response and different results will be achieved.

The amount of attention which the patient receives during the study (by the "Hawthorne effect") affects placebo response. Improved response comes with increased attention as shown by sick elderly patients whose condition usually improves if nurses visit regularly.

Work with morphine showed a placebo response of about 35% in a large group of patients, and some authorities believe that placebo reactors can be identified. There is an argument that these should be discovered and then excluded from clinical trials. However, although 35% of patients respond to placebo on average, it is not necessarily the same ones each time. Indeed placebo response may sometimes be as high as 75 – 80%.

In general the placebo response tends to tail off with time, and this effect may be noted in a long-term study.

Using placebo in double blind studies

Placebo may be used to enable a study comparing two drugs with different dose forms (eg. tablets and capsules) to be conducted in a double blind manner. For example, assume that a capsule and a tablet will be compared. In order to make the study double blind, each time a patient has to take a dose of study medication, they have to take one capsule and one tablet (Figure 5). Therefore, patients who have been allocated to treatment with the tablets (Group A) will take one active tablet and one placebo capsule, whilst those patients who have been allocated to treatment with the capsule (Group B) will take one active capsule and one placebo tablet. By using this technique, neither the patient nor the investigator is aware of which active medication the patient is receiving. This is a very common technique in comparative clinical trials and is called the *"double dummy technique"*.

Payment in clinical trials

It is usual that the investigator in a clinical trial receives a fee for his services. The size of the fee is variable and is often calculated

FIGURE 5. Double dummy design.

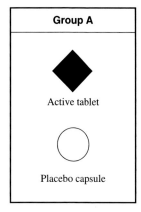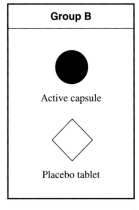

Both groups take a tablet and a capsule but only one is active.

on a cost per patient basis rather than by offering a general "unconditional" grant. Overheads are often charged by hospitals, pharmacies and laboratories who participate in a trial. Healthy volunteers are also paid for taking part in Phase I studies, although the level of remuneration should be modest. It should be noted that patients are not paid for taking part in clinical trials, but in exceptional circumstances assistance may be offered with travelling expenses.

Payments to doctors who take part in trials is a controversial issue. Some groups feel that "per-capita" payments are unethical as they encourage investigators to enter unsuitable patients in trials for financial gain. On the other hand, a company who makes a grant to an investigator may end up paying out large sums of money and getting little or nothing in return. Trial payments are often used to subsidise other research activities, for buying equipment or as travel funds, but frequently they are retained as private income by the investigator. There are no specific rules about this.

Payments are determined for each trial and their magnitude depends greatly on the nature of the study and the therapeutic area.

MEASUREMENT IN CLINICAL TRIALS

Measuring efficacy

The effectiveness of treatment is measured by comparing the condition of the patient before treatment with the condition after treatment. Intermediate assessments may also be undertaken whilst treatment is in progress to determine the speed of improvement in the patient's condition.

Numerous methods exist to determine the improvement and deterioration of the patient. Many are subjective such as questionnaires and rating scales, whilst on some occasions it is possible to make objective determinations by measuring, for example, blood pressure, heart rate and respiratory flow rate using equipment which produces numerical values which can be recorded. Objective determinations are most likely to show differences between baseline and the end of treatment, because subjective measures tend to have much greater variability in their interpretation.

One of the most commonly used questionnaires is the Hamilton Depression Rating Scale which can be used to measure the severity of a patient's depression. Here the doctor will ask the patient a number of questions about how they feel and the symptoms they experience; the doctor will then score the response according to severity on a numerical scale. The score from each question is added up to give a total score which can be compared before and after treatment to see how the patient has responded. There are many similar questionnaires in current use covering other therapeutic areas.

Rating scales often take the form of four- or five-point scales. For example, in the measurement of the severity of pain a patient can be asked to grade their pain as absent (no pain), mild, moderate or severe. This scale has four categories; a fifth may be

---

FIGURE 6. A categorical rating scale.

Absent ☐   Mild ☐   Moderate ☐   Severe ☑   Very Severe ☐

---

added such as "very severe" in an attempt to make the scale more sensitive (Figure 6).

A further example of a rating scale is the visual analogue scale (VAS). This is traditionally a line of 100 mm in length where each end represents an extreme of the condition being assessed. For example, if you are trying to assess how well a patient slept, the left hand end would be labelled "no sleep at all" whilst the right hand end of the line would be labelled "best sleep ever experienced" (Figure 7). The patient would be asked to rate how he/she slept last night and would make a single mark on the line to represent this. The distance from the left hand end to the mark made by the patient would then be measured and this would be the value recorded to represent how the patient slept. It can be seen therefore that a VAS is a way of allocating a numerical value to a subjective feeling.

Whichever measure of efficacy is selected, care must be taken to ensure that the method is reliable, valid and, more importantly, likely to be suitable to show a difference between before and after treatment findings as well as differences between treatments. Many routine clinical assessments are only useful for diagnosing diseases and are

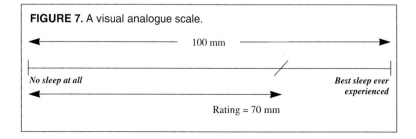

FIGURE 7. A visual analogue scale.

100 mm

No sleep at all   *Best sleep ever experienced*

Rating = 70 mm

not sensitive enough to measure reliable changes in a patient's condition. A statistician should be consulted early in the planning of a trial in order that the best assessment methods may be chosen.

A confounding factor in the measurement of efficacy is the placebo response; in the development of a new drug it is important to show that the active drug is more effective than treatment with placebo. This is not always easy and this is the downfall of many new compounds. It is also important to compare the effectiveness of new drugs with those already available, including the market leader; this is information that both the regulatory authorities and the prescriber will want to consider.

Measurements of efficacy are usually divided into primary measures (ie. the most important measure on which most emphasis is placed) and secondary measures (ie. those which are important and may be used to support the results of the primary measures).

Measuring safety

The most common measures of safety are recording vital signs, blood and urine tests and adverse events. Laboratory tests may be undertaken to determine how well the major organs of the body are functioning, in particular the liver, heart and kidneys. Enzymes and substances in the blood may increase or decrease in level and these give sensitive and early guides to malfunction which may be caused by a new drug, as well as giving useful clinical information about the patient's general condition. Vital signs include regular measurement of blood pressure, heart rate, temperature and weight; the effect of taking a new treatment on these parameters is an important safety measure. Adverse events are, perhaps, the most reliable measure of the tolerability of a treatment and are described in more detail below.

Patient protection is important and the measurements of safety undertaken in a clinical trial must demonstrate that the new compound has a tolerable level of side effects, particularly when compared with products already on the market.

Adverse events

● *Definition*

Adverse events (AEs) are all undesirable experiences occurring to a subject during a clinical trial, whether or not they are related to the investigational product. When an *adverse event* has been assessed and there are reasonable grounds for suspecting that it is related to the treatment under investigation, it becomes an *adverse drug reaction* (ADR). Adverse event recording is an important measure of drug safety and treatment tolerability.

In all clinical trials, the investigator is called upon to assess the causality of any adverse event. Usually four categories are used to describe the relationship with treatment: namely definite, probably, possibly and not-assessable. The assessment of causality is rather arbitrary in most cases, with the investigator using his clinical judgement and knowledge of the investigational products.

● *Seriousness of the event*

Adverse events can be divided into two types: serious and non-serious (often termed trivial). It is a requirement that investigators report serious adverse events immediately, by telephone, to the sponsor of the study. By definition, serious events are those that are fatal or life threatening, disabling, congenital abnormalities, events that result in hospitalisation as an in-patient and those that prolong the stay in hospital. The occurrence of malignancy, pregnancy and overdose would be deemed to be serious events. Other significant medical events can also be considered to be serious adverse events. The sponsor of the study will document all serious adverse events with special attention, dealing with matters rapidly and carefully before transmitting the information gathered to the regulatory authority. A separate report form is often provided with the CRF for recording the details of a serious adverse event.

Non-serious or trivial events should be recorded in the appropriate section of the patient's CRF, which is provided by the sponsor. These events will be evaluated by the study monitor as the trial progresses and eventually summarised in the Final Report produced at the end of the study.

● *Is the event unexpected?*
Adverse events that have been reported in previous trials are usually described in the "Investigator Brochure" (a comprehensive description of the test product and its characteristics). Events that have not been reported previously, and those that have been reported but then occur more frequently or more severely, are termed "unexpected".

● *Reporting requirements*
Serious, unexpected adverse drug reactions need to be reported to the regulatory authorities, by the sponsor, within 15 days of receiving the report (7 days if fatal event). The Ethics Committee who approved the study also need to be informed of these events.

● *Duration of the event*
The duration of all adverse events needs to be recorded. Usually the investigator is asked to record duration as the number of days or hours, together with a start date. It is also important to report that the event resolved, spontaneously or after treatment, or continued. Some adverse events are transient and occur for only a short time after commencing treatment; others may continue from onset of treatment until stopping the medication.

● *Severity of the event*
The severity of the event and its seriousness are often confused. Serious events have been defined above; it is quite possible to have a severe event which does not fall into the serious category, eg. headache. This would be described as a non-serious event, unless it

resulted in hospitalisation. The patient may, however, suffer from a severe headache which lasts for some days. This event would be recorded in the CRF but telephone contact with the study monitor would not be deemed necessary. The event should, however, be discussed with the monitor at his/her next visit to the investigator.

The severity of the adverse event is usually categorised as "mild, moderate or severe". Occasionally, "very severe" is an additional category. The investigator should use his clinical judgement to evaluate severity. As a guideline, a mild event is unlikely to interfere with the patient's daily activities whilst a severe one may well result in the patient taking a day off work or other inconvenience.

● *Treatment and outcome*
Sometimes the adverse event may require treatment with a drug. Before prescribing, the investigator must take note of any excluded drugs, as defined in the study protocol; if a drug must be given that is excluded, then the patient has to be withdrawn from the study and the reasons recorded in the patient's CRF. If the desired treatment is permitted then the investigator should record the use of concomitant medication in the appropriate section in the CRF. Details of dose, route, duration and reason for treatment should be given.

In all cases the outcome of the event should be recorded. This may simply mean classifying the event as "resolved spontaneously", "resolved after treatment" or "unresolved".

In recent years the removal of drugs from the market due to a high incidence of unacceptable or unwanted side effects has emphasised the need for accurate and reliable reporting of adverse events in clinical trials. It is the responsibility of investigators to fully document all adverse events which occur in trials they undertake. It is also important for the sponsor of trials, through its monitors, to ensure that all adverse events are properly documented.

2

The critical path of the clinical trial

<table>
<tr><td>INTRODUCTION</td></tr>
</table>

Increasing costs and regulatory requirements needing more and more clinical research in order to achieve drug registration demand that clinical trials are well planned and efficiently executed to rigorous timescales. It is important, therefore, to fully understand the critical path of the clinical trial and the action required at each stage to minimise delays. Collaboration with colleagues within the company is essential; delays often occur due to lack of information and advance notice of impending requirements. Delays caused by third parties, such as Ethics Committees and regulatory authorities, can be minimised by careful assessment of documentation needs and meeting dates before submission.

The key to the success of the clinical trial is the selection of the study investigator. Whether carried out in hospital or general practice, high quality studies are usually performed by well motivated, diligent trialists. A high regard for ethics and legal requirements is essential at all times and a good working knowledge of Good Clinical Practice (GCP) Guidelines is important for all involved in the trial.

Overall, understanding and anticipating the problems arising in the critical path of the clinical trial is vital to the success of the study. Collaboration, with efficient exchange of information, will ensure that trials are completed efficiently and on time. This chapter reviews the stages involved in the critical path of a clinical trial and suggests how some of the commonly occurring problems may be avoided.

FIGURE 8. The critical path of the clinical trial.

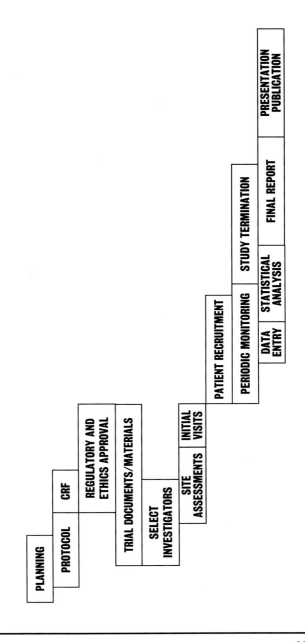

STAGES OF THE CLINICAL TRIAL

Let us now examine the stages which make up the critical path of a clinical trial performed in the UK.

The typical path of a clinical trial is shown in Figure 8. This path may be applied to most situations. All sections represent independent courses of action.

To minimise the time taken to undertake a study

- the processes involved in each section should be carefully reviewed and made as efficient as possible
- deadlines should be placed on the completion of each task, with constant review and revision as the study progresses
- all personnel involved in the study must be kept fully informed at each review stage; adequate information exchange by parties involved in the path will ensure efficient completion of the study.

Planning

In the past, many studies have been undertaken by pharmaceutical companies without careful planning, and in particular without due regard for regulatory requirements and marketing strategy. In recent years, however, the co-ordination of research plans by project teams has had a major influence on the effectiveness of the clinical trial programme to obtain product licences in shorter timescales and support subsequent marketing plans. The planning of clinical studies should therefore be a co-ordinated effort by representatives of the medical department, usually the Medical Adviser and Clinical Research Associate responsible for the project, a statistician, the trials supplies pharmacist, a member of the data management team, a representative of the Regulatory Affairs Department and the Product Manager from the marketing department. Agreement on the course of action to be taken is essential. Careful estimates of time and cost should be prepared against agreed time schedules. The prioritisation of projects should be undertaken at this stage and important, high priority studies should be identified; potential problems, their prevention and solution should be anticipated in order that agreed deadlines may be adhered to. Contingency plans should be discussed.

Although the project team oversees each study, it is usually the responsibility of the trial monitor to ensure that each stage of the trial is successfully completed.

The study protocol

Usually, the first draft of the protocol is prepared by the Clinical Research Associate or Medical Adviser responsible for setting up the study.

Once this has been prepared, internal review of the document should be undertaken; the comments of the statistician should be particularly noted. Comments should be incorporated into the second revision. At this stage, potential investigators or members of a steering committee, set up to oversee and advise on study conduct, should be invited to advise on the suitability of the protocol. It is commonly the case that companies do not wish to allow investigators to make comments on the protocol; this is perhaps unfair and may ultimately lead to inefficient patient recruitment. Although the company may wish to stipulate trial design, dosage, treatment duration and assessment methods, it is important that the investigator and company, together, review the inclusion and exclusion criteria relating to the study population and the practical aspects of undertaking the study. In a multicentre study, a representative steering committee of two or three investigators can be empowered to act on behalf of the whole investigator panel in order to improve the overall practicability of the study.

Delays in the planning and finalisation of the study protocol may be minimised by setting a deadline for the receipt of comments and, if necessary, demonstrating the effect of delay on the overall critical path of the study. Agreement of priorities is absolutely essential in order to avoid delays in approval. As soon as the protocol has been finalised, but not until, it may be submitted for Ethics Committee and regulatory approval.

Case record forms

The case record forms (CRFs) should be prepared after the final draft of the protocol has been prepared. Although time may be saved at the data entry stage of the study by well designed record forms, the first priority should always be to ensure their easy and foolproof completion by the investigator. For this reason, it is preferable that input from the investigator is obtained. Proper CRF design is essential for the success of any study. Good CRF design will also reduce overall monitoring time in relation to checking and correction, thus making the study more cost effective.

Ethics and regulatory affairs

In the early part of the trial ethics and regulatory affairs are the main areas for delay; this is usually outside the direct control of the sponsoring company. However, adequate preparation, forward planning and collaboration can minimise any delay in the approval of a study.

In the planning stages of the study, potentially suitable investigators should be identified and principal investigators appointed. These may form the basis of the steering committee for the study, provide investigators' names for submission to the regulatory authorities and allow early submission of the final protocol to an independent Ethics Committee for approval. It is essential that approval is obtained from the Ethics Committee at each centre (the institutional review board (IRB) in the USA), and careful checking should be undertaken to ensure that the IRB is properly constituted according to Federal (ie. US) or GCP rules.

Prior to the finalisation of the protocol, and as early as possible in the critical path of the study, the requirements of the Ethics Committee/IRB, particularly with regard to the documentation, dates of the next meeting, procedure for submission and so on, should be determined to minimise any subsequent delay. The date of the next meeting of the committee is an important constraint on the critical path of the study and, where possible, all early planning deadlines should fall into line with this. Sufficient time should be allowed in the critical path for Ethics Committee/IRB approval. In general, it is unlikely that approval will be obtained within one month; on average one or two months elapse before the procedure is finalised. In some countries, it is not unknown for approval to take as long as six months to one year; if that is the case the monitor should consider the wisdom of selecting that particular centre for the study. The terms of re-approval for long studies should also be considered.

It is worthy of note that at the time of writing few Ethics Committees in Europe are properly constituted, as defined by various GCP Guidelines. This matter should be addressed when planning a study. Additionally, the European Community Guidelines for GCP require Ethics Committees to play a much greater role in the clinical trial than currently is the case.

Early notification of impending clinical trials is appreciated by the Regulatory Affairs Department. This will enable staff to plan the preparation of an application to appropriate authorities for regulatory approval to commence the study. Regulatory approval has been discussed in more detail in Chapter 1.

With careful planning, regular exchange of information and collaboration, delays in the critical path caused by Ethics Committee/IRB approval and regulatory approval can be kept to a minimum.

Selection of investigators

Whilst the protocol is in the stages of finalisation, potential investigators should be identified. The selection of good investigators is crucial to the success of any study. Those already known to the company and who have a reliable previous record regarding clinical research are to be preferred. Random mailings are rarely effective when establishing an investigator panel de novo; my own experiences show that positive replies to letters inviting doctors to participate may be in the order of 1 in 10 or even as low as 1 in 20. Recommendations from colleagues, other investigators and representatives and review of published literature may be used to identify investigators. One simple measure of suitability as an investigator is "The Correspondence Test". Write a letter to the potential investigator, requesting information, and evaluate their response. Some will not reply and will need chasing: these, I suggest, may not be the best investigators subsequently. The best investigators are likely to be those that respond in a reasonable amount of time, providing the information you have requested. The true effectiveness of an investigator can only be assessed at the end of each study and even those who have performed well previously may fail on another occasion.

A copy of the curriculum vitae of each investigator and co-investigator should be obtained to confirm that they are appropriately qualified and are "academically suitable" for taking part in the study. Often investigators do not have up-to-date CVs and the company can help by providing a standard form for completion or indeed by making good use of information in the Medical Directory. The names of staff assisting the investigator, for example the pharmacist, technicians and study nurse, should also be obtained. Some regulatory authorities keep a list of unsuitable investigators and their opinion could be sought if in doubt.

Site assessment and pre-study briefing

Site assessment should be performed to ensure that selected investigators have the necessary facilities, potential number of patients, time, motivation and resources to undertake the study. Only a visit by the study monitor can confirm this. Site assessment visits can be made as soon as an investigator has been identified. For a multicentre study, this may be a lengthy task and should be started as soon as possible in the trial critical path so as to avoid later delays. All study centres should be visited.

The pre-study briefing may be undertaken in groups or individually. Detailed discussion of the type of patient to be recruited, the completion of the record forms and administrative procedures to be followed should be carried out. Some evaluation of the investigator's understanding of the study protocol, his or her obligations during the study and the likely recruitment rate should be performed. Targets for patient recruitment should be agreed. Other matters, such as verification of data obtained in the study and payments must be discussed, and a course of action agreed, before the study commences.

Study materials

The preparation and printing of study documents such as consent forms, patient information packs, case record forms and investigator brochures should be undertaken as early as possible in the path of the study. Try to inform the pharmacist in the trial supplies department as soon as possible about the quantity of medication required and how the materials are to be packed and labelled so that orders can be placed for the required items. Many trials are held up as a result of delays in preparation of the trial materials; on most occasions this arises as a result of poor communication and exchange of information.

The six stages in the critical path described above are largely under the control of the pharmaceutical company and its staff, with the exception of the Ethics Committee/IRB and regulatory authority. Delays caused in the planning and preparation of the study are often the result of an excessive workload and inadequate identification and management of priorities. It is important, when planning a study, that personnel at all levels are in agreement with time schedules and strategy; the critical path analysis may then be used to demonstrate the effect of any delays on the overall time schedule of the study.

Early delays may have a significant effect on the motivation of the investigator. Often unaware of the internal administrative tasks to be performed once a study protocol has been finalised, the investigator is usually keen to start patient recruitment. Frequent contact with the investigator by the monitor is important at this stage to maintain enthusiasm and motivation; lengthy delays leading up to the start of patient recruitment can only have a negative effect on the critical path of the study. The period between protocol finalisation and the start of patient recruitment, ie. the time spent waiting for various approvals and trial materials, may be effectively used by the investigator to identify suitable patients or to determine, more accurately, the anticipated recruitment rate by application of the study inclusion and exclusion criteria to patients passing thorough his clinics. This has a positive effect on the investigator's motivation.

Once ethics and regulatory approval have been received, recruitment of patients to the study may begin.

Patient recruitment

Providing prediction of suitable patients has been accurate and the study protocol is appropriate, particularly with regard to the inclusion and exclusion of patients, then the process of patient recruitment should be straightforward.

Unfortunately poor recruitment is a common problem and is usually due to inaccurate prediction of the number of patients an investigator can enter. When questioned, investigators usually predict the total number of patients with a particular condition known to them, forgetting that inclusion/exclusion criteria make some of these unsuitable and the fact that some patients will not wish to participate in the study. As few as 50 – 60% of initially predicted patients may actually enter the study, causing a shortfall against the total planned number required.

Many investigators like to enter a single patient in the early stages of the study to "bench test" the methodology and protocol. Careful monitoring of patient recruitment should be carried out, especially when the first few enter the study, to ensure that the study protocol is being properly followed and the record forms are correctly completed.

Investigators who do not enter patients soon after the start of recruitment should be carefully evaluated; further reasons for poor recruitment often include misinterpretation of entry criteria in the planning stages of the study, too rigorous inclusion criteria, and lack of interest, motivation, time and resources.

In general, investigators should try to establish special clinics for patients in clinical trials. This is relatively easy for studies in hypertension, hay fever and so on. For some conditions, however, this is not possible, for example infections and acutely painful indications, where attendance at a regular surgery is the only way to identify suitable patients.

Recruitment may be improved by scanning an age-sex register and writing to potentially suitable patients (eg. those with menopausal symptoms), having a poster in the surgery offering a special study clinic (eg. a hypertension or hay fever clinic) or screening all patients who enter the surgery.

No pressure must be placed on patients to take part in a study and their informed consent must always be obtained before they are entered. Furthermore, no undue pressure should be placed on the investigator to recruit patients to the study as this increases the likelihood of entering patients in default of the study protocol.

Overall, effective patient recruitment should be undertaken in approximately three to six months. Longer recruitment periods fail to "concentrate the mind" in the early stages and complacency may set in. In addition, investigators may become demotivated if the study is too long and their attentions may move towards new projects. The number of centres required and the number of patients per centre should be carefully determined with this in mind, including an overage for dropouts, withdrawals and unsuitable patients; sufficient number of centres should be kept in reserve in case unforeseen problems occur once recruitment has started.

Periodic monitoring

During the study, the monitor should visit each investigator every four to eight weeks, depending on the length of the study, to check on study progress. Patient entry in accordance with the study protocol should be checked, as should the completion of the CRFs. All pharmaceutical companies should have Standard Operating Procedures describing how frequently the monitor should visit each investigational site, together with a description of the checks and tasks that should be performed at each visit. If the study is conducted according to GCP Guidelines, validation checks on the data collected by the investigator should be performed. Good Clinical Practice guidelines now require the monitor to perform "direct source data verification". This is where the monitor compares data written in the CRF with source data (eg. patient files, print-outs of laboratory results and automated instruments, etc). This process is to check the reliability of data collected. The monitor also checks the CRF to ensure it has been fully completed and the data are legible. All alterations and errors in the CRF need to be initialled and dated by the investigator.

Completed and checked record forms may be collected by the monitor at each visit and passed on to the data monitor for further checking before the process of data entry.

To conserve time, data entry may be undertaken whilst the study is in progress. This also enables testing and verification of the database in plenty of time to meet future deadlines.

Study termination

As each centre completes the study, all remaining trial materials, including unused medication, used patient packs, record forms, code breaking envelopes and other documents, should be collected by the monitor. The investigator should retain consent forms and the register of names of patients who took part in the study, as well as copies of study results, the protocol and correspondence. The study termination phase may also include clarification of inconsistencies and missing data revealed as a result of data monitoring and quality assurance.

If the trial monitors have been diligent during the study and have checked CRFs as the study progressed, delays in data management at the end of the study should be minimal.

Data entry and statistical analysis

Early involvement of the statistician in study planning should ensure that the process of data entry is undertaken speedily and effectively once the study has finished. Delays in data entry are often the result of lack of communication regarding the date CRFs will be available, poor CRF design giving rise to data entry difficulties and poor monitoring giving rise to numerous queries requiring attention before the database is complete.

The project team should ensure that the statistician has allocated time to the project as data become available. A source of great irritation to investigators and monitors alike is the long delay in receiving study results, especially if the investigator has been "hurried along" to meet deadlines only for the analysis to take 12 months to perform. Collaboration, progress reports during the study and co-operation by all parties can help avoid unnecessary delay at the end of the study. Most time is taken up in data entry; the analysis and preparation of the statistical report is relatively quick if a computerised database is set up.

Quality assurance checks should be made at all stages of data entry and analysis. Double data entry helps minimise errors and a manual check on a certain percentage of the data, $10 - 20\%$, is usually performed by the statistician before final analysis.

Two to three months is typically the time necessary for data entry and analysis, depending on the size and complexity of the study. Of this period, only two or three weeks should be required for statistical analysis and report production.

The Final Report

The Final Report is prepared from the protocol, record forms and statistical report and is the comprehensive description of the methods and results of the study, interpretation of the findings, and tabulations and full listings of all data collected. The Final Report may be written in addition to the statistical report or fully integrated with it as a single document.

The time taken to write the Final Report is relatively short. Delays are usually caused by the need for numerous in-house reviews and approval. The investigator should also be asked to review the Final Report and to show his approval of the final document by signature.

For studies on drugs not yet licensed, data presented in the Final Report are likely to be submitted to the regulatory authorities to support a product licence application. In any event, the results will be reported to the authorities for information purposes. It is vital, therefore, that all patients entered into the study are accounted for and no inconsistencies occur between tables and text.

The final stages of the critical path of the study are those of preparing a paper for publication and the presentation of the study at a meeting or congress, unless the data obtained need to remain confidential. Publication times can be considerably shortened by submission to journals with a rapid turnover, such as the *British Journal of Clinical Research* and the *European Journal of Clinical Research,* where publication is achieved only 21 days after acceptance. This ensures the results of the study are used effectively whilst the data are still current. Sometimes publication in highly prestigious medical journals is required but this can often take many months or years to achieve.

From planning to Final Report, a typical clinical trial can be expected to take from 12 to 24 months to complete. Some trials with long treatment periods obviously take much longer whilst single dose studies can be completed much more quickly.

3

Good clinical practice

The need for good clinical practice

The standard of clinical research between countries worldwide is highly variable. For many years the USA has claimed to be the flagship for quality and reliability of data. This has arisen as a result of stringent rules and regulations regarding the conduct of companies, monitors and investigators performing clinical trials. The void in quality was so great that the regulatory body in the USA responsible for the approval of product licence applications, the Food and Drug Administration (FDA), would not accept some data collected outside the USA as principal evidence of a drug's safety and efficacy; in fact, review bodies determined that the quality of "foreign" data was unreliable because:

- protocols were not detailed enough to ensure that data were properly collected
- CRFs were badly designed
- inadequate records regarding the conduct of the study were kept
- investigators were not monitored closely enough
- no checks on the reliability of data were performed
- inappropriate methods of analysis were used.

Indeed, some studies in the UK have been performed by post: the investigator was never visited, data were never checked and the reliability of the study was never questioned. It then emerged that, in a number of cases in the UK, investigators had made up results or entered data in the CRFs that had been invented. Clinical trial fraud was found to be a worldwide problem. Other deficiencies included recruitment of patients without their consent, failure to report adverse events, investigators breaking the drug code to improve the results, studies performed without Ethics Committee approval, and so on. These occurrences, together with the "unintentional errors" that inevitably occur during the course of a clinical trial, suggest that data collected in some trials were truly unreliable and that many studies in the past may have indeed been improperly conducted.

In order to improve the conduct of studies and the quality of data collected, the UK and many other European countries introduced guidelines, in the mid-to-late 1980s, to improve research standards resembling those used in the USA, called Good Clinical Practice (GCP).

What is Good Clinical Practice (GCP)?

> *A standard for the design, conduct, performance, monitoring, auditing, recording, analyses and reporting of clinical trials that provides assurance that the data and reported results are credible and accurate, and that the rights, integrity and confidentiality of trial subjects are protected.*
>
> ICH GCP Glossary 1.24

Good Clinical Practice (GCP) details the quality processes required in the conduct of clinical trials. In most countries world-wide, GCP is a legal requirement and if these rules are not followed the Boards of Health who make decisions about the licensing of a new product will reject the clinical trial data submitted as it may be unreliable. This might also damage the research credibility of the investigator and centre. It is vital, therefore, that all investigators who undertake clinical trials have a thorough working knowledge of the GCP requirements and adhere to them.

GCP helps to ensure that subjects (healthy volunteers or patients as appropriate) are appropriately protected during the course of a clinical trial: it ensures that written informed consent is properly obtained and that each trial has the approval of an independent Ethics Committee before the study commences. In addition, implementation of GCP prevents studies with improper designs or insufficient sample sizes from being performed. An important part of GCP is the collection and maintenance of documents in the trial that demonstrate that all the GCP requirements have been undertaken.

GCP ensures that:
● Subjects are properly protected in the studies
● Studies are based on good science, are well designed and properly analysed
● The study procedures are properly undertaken and documented.

If GCP is not followed:
● The subjects who take part may be at risk
● The data collected may be unreliable
● The study might be rejected by the Boards of Health.

Harmonisation of GCP?

GCP was born in the USA in the mid 1970s when the Food & Drug Administration (FDA) implemented guidelines for clinical investigators; this was followed by rigorous investigational new drug (IND) procedures which have been modified over the years to the version that is in force today. Strict implementation of the new regulations in the USA led to the FDA rejecting data from other countries; it considered the data to be substandard. This meant that a company who wanted to market a drug in the USA had to repeat its clinical research in accordance with the IND regulations before it would be accepted.

This forced a review of procedures in other countries and led to the birth of various national GCPs, eventually followed by a set of European GCP guidelines, developed by the member states and implemented in 1990. Most European companies have been working in accordance with these GCPs.

There were differences, however, in GCP procedures in Europe, USA and the third large pharmaceutical market, Japan, who developed their own GCPs in 1991. These differences meant that the data collected in one region would not be accepted automatically by another region, even though it might have been performed in accordance with local GCP requirements.

As a result, the regulatory authorities and representatives of the pharmaceutical companies in the USA, Europe and Japan, together with observers from Scandinavia, Australia, Canada and the WHO, held a series of meetings to develop a set of GCPs that would be universally accepted.

In May 1996, the ICH GCPs were finalised and these have now become the standard by which all clinical trials have to be performed in order to achieve universal recognition [1].

The European regulatory authorities (CPMP) have instructed that all trials performed in Europe (starting 1 January 1997) for regulatory purposes must be performed in accordance with the ICH GCP guidelines and these have now superseded previous European GCPs. A Directive will be implemented sometime in 1997 to make ICH GCPs a legal requirement and this will then be incorporated into the national law of EU member states. The ICH GCPs were reproduced in the US Federal Register in May 1997 and the FDA expect all trials conducted outside of the US and used to support an application for marketing authorisation (NDA, new drug application) to be conducted in accordance with these if not already performed to IND Regulations. Japan implemented the ICH GCPs in April 1997.

Standard Operating Procedures

In response to GCP guidelines, each company is required to prepare and implement a set of Standard Operating Procedures (SOPs). These specify, in detail, how the company will undertake its clinical research projects in accordance with the GCP rules. Writing the SOPs is very difficult; once finalised and accepted, the company must operate in accordance with the specified methods, and, in the absence of a good reason to deviate, the acceptability of a research project, and hence subsequent product licence applications, may be jeopardised if the house rules are not followed. SOPs override all GCP guidelines.

It is important, therefore, that staff participating in a clinical trial have read and are familiar with the SOPs relating to their job function. It cannot be over-emphasised that strict adherence to SOPs is essential.

Responsibilities

It is important that all professional staff undertaking a trial to GCP standards share the responsibility of "getting things right". The role of the secretary/administrator is very important; it is insufficient to expect that a 9 am to 5 pm role sheds any responsibility for performing studies to GCP. In fact, the secretary/administrator should be extremely diligent in performing clinical research duties. GCP is based on sound documentation and administration; the trial files, often maintained by the secretary, are one of the most important parts of GCP.

With the introduction of GCP many experienced staff have had to modify their usual working procedures. This inevitably has caused some resentment. GCP has the advantage of harmonising working procedures within a company and whilst there is still room for some personal methods, the overall effect is greater efficiency and less margin for errors to occur – providing SOPs are followed by all staff.

OUTLINE OF ICH GOOD CLINICAL PRACTICE GUIDELINES

Protection of trial subjects and consultation of Ethics Committees

- All studies must be conducted in accordance with the current revision of the Declaration of Helsinki (South Africa, October 1996; Appended). This ensures that the individual's rights are protected and that subjects give consent to take part in a clinical study. In addition, subjects can withdraw from studies at any time without giving a reason and such withdrawal does not prejudice any future medical treatment.

- All clinical trial protocols must be submitted to and approved by an Independent Ethics Committee before a study can begin. The Ethics Committee will ensure that the study is ethical and that the subject's rights are protected. Subjects must be informed that they are being asked to take part in a research study. Full information about the study and the drug which is to be tested must be provided to each subject. This information should be provided verbally and in writing.

- Consent must be obtained from each subject before any study procedures are undertaken. A total of 20 items of information must be presented to the subject in writing and verbally. The Ethics Committee will review the written information sheet and the consent form that is to be used in the study. It will also ensure that subjects are aware of any compensation in the event of injury or death, and that the sponsor provides indemnity insurance to cover the liability of the investigator and the sponsor in the event of any untoward event arising as a result of a subject taking part in the study.

With regard to Ethics Committees, the ICH GCP Guidelines ask that the suitability of the investigator (eg. experience, staff and equipment) to undertake the study in question is confirmed. If not, the Ethics Committee may decide that it would be unethical to proceed with the study at that site.

Before entering a study, each subject must receive full information about the nature of the test drug and the study and must be given an opportunity to ask questions about any aspect of the trial. An information sheet should also be provided for each subject. If the subject still wishes to participate in the study then he or she will be asked to sign and date the consent form which is also countersigned and dated by the investigator. In some countries, written informed consent is not the local practice and in these situations subjects can give verbal consent to take part in a trial. Under these circumstances, the consent form will usually be signed and dated by the investigator and also by a witness who was present during the whole consent procedure, and who can verify that the subject was given full information and had an opportunity to ask questions and gave free verbal consent to study participation.

Responsibilities

The responsibilities in the study are shared between the sponsor (usually the pharmaceutical company or contract research organisation), the monitor and the investigator and these are summarised below.

Sponsor's responsibilities
- To establish detailed SOPs
- To prepare the study protocol (and obtain investigator agreement)

- To select appropriate investigators
- To conduct a pre-study site inspection
- To provide information on the test drug in an Investigator's Brochure (which should be updated regularly)
- To obtain regulatory approval for the study
- To ensure that the protocol is submitted for ethics approval
- To provide clinical trial supplies manufactured to Good Manufacturing Practice (GMP) standards
- To report any serious unexpected adverse reactions to the Ethics Committee and to the regulatory authority
- To prepare a comprehensive Final Report in accordance with ICH Guidelines
- To provide adequate compensation in case of injury or death and to provide indemnification insurance for the investigator (and if necessary the area health authority)
- To agree with the investigator on the policies regarding data handling, reporting of results and publication of study data
- To validate all systems for data handling.

Monitor's responsibilities
- To act as the principal communication link between the sponsor and the investigator
- To comply with the company's SOPs
- To be familiar with the test product, the study protocol, CRFs, consent form, SOPs, GCP and regulatory requirements
- To visit the investigator before, during and after completion of the trial to check adherence to protocol, ensure that all data are recorded accurately and to validate that informed consent was obtained from all patients before undergoing any trial procedures
- To ensure that the trial site has the facilities and the staff required to undertake the trial
- To ensure that all the investigator's staff have been adequately informed about the study and that they comply with the procedures laid down in the study protocol

- To check CRF entries against source documents by using direct source data verification, and to inform the investigator of any errors or omissions
- To check that drug storage, dispensing and return and documentation of the supply of study drug(s) are safe and appropriate and in accordance with local regulations
- To assist the investigator in any notification or application procedure that may be required in order to conduct the study
- To submit a written report to the sponsor after each site visit and suitable contact reports after telephone calls and other contacts.

Investigator's responsibilities

- To understand the properties of the investigational drug as described in the Investigator's Brochure
- To ensure that sufficient time and resources are devoted to the conduct of the trial
- To provide retrospective data on the numbers of patients who would have satisfied the proposed entry criteria for the study over a given time period to determine whether the required recruitment rate can be met
- To provide a current curriculum vitae
- To maintain a log of study personnel
- To agree to comply with the protocol and the principles of GCP
- To submit the protocol to the local Ethics Committee for approval
- To obtain informed consent from all subjects taking part in the trial
- To keep a log of subjects screened and details of those who enter the study
- To collect, record and report data correctly
- To notify the sponsor and, when applicable, the Ethics Committee regarding the occurrence of any serious adverse events
- To make all data available to the sponsor, the monitor or relevant authorities for verification, audit or inspection purposes

- To agree on the content of the Final Report
- To ensure that the confidentiality of all information about subjects, as well as the information that is supplied by the sponsor, is respected by all persons involved in the study
- To make all medical decisions regarding subjects in the study.

Data handling

● *Data recording*

The investigator is responsible for ensuring that the observations and findings noted in a study are recorded correctly and accurately in the CRFs. All corrections made on CRFs or elsewhere in the hard copy raw data must be made in a way which does not obscure the original entry: a single line should be drawn through the erroneous data and the correct data inserted with the reason for the correction. The correction should be dated and initialled by the investigator. Correcting fluids should never be used.

Laboratory values with the normal reference ranges should always be recorded on the CRF or attached to it. Values outside a clinically accepted reference range or values that differ importantly from previous values must be evaluated and commented upon by the investigator.

The monitor should visit the investigator at regular intervals during the study to review the data contained in the CRF. The purpose of these visits is to correct errors and to compare the data contained in the CRF with the source data usually contained in the patient's medical notes. In addition, the monitor must take appropriate measures to avoid overlooking missing data or logical inconsistencies.

Entry to a computerised data system is acceptable. However, when electronic data handling systems (or remote electronic data entry) are used, SOPs must be established. The computer system used should be designed to allow data to be corrected after loading and any such correction must appear in the audit file. Only authorised persons are allowed to change data once it has been entered into the computer system. If trial data are entered into a computer there must be adequate safeguards to ensure the validity of these data, including a signed data print-out and back-up records. If data are altered during processing, the alteration must be documented.

● *Archiving*

The investigator must keep trial documentation, including the identification codes for patients participating in clinical trials, until instructed by the sponsor that they are no longer required. Patient files and other source data must be kept for the maximum period of time permitted by the hospital, institution or private practice. The investigator must ensure that these important documents are not destroyed prematurely. Sponsors are required to retain trial documents until 2 years after the last marketing authorisation in the ICH region. This is an undefined period. In practice, the sponsor (or the subsequent owner of the product) usually retains all documentation pertaining to the trial for the lifetime of the product.

Archived data may be held on microfiche or electronic record, provided that a back-up exists and that hard copy can be obtained from it if required. Many companies now have off-site storage facilities where documents are kept away from light in temperature controlled, fire-proof surroundings.

Statistics

A biostatistician should be involved in many aspects of the study. These include the following:
- ● trial design
- ● assessing the power of the study (that is the likelihood of showing a difference between treatments)
- ● calculating the number of patients needed to detect a statistical difference

- preparation of the statistical analysis plan which should be included in the study protocol detailing how the results will be analysed at the end of the trial
- involvement in measures taken to avoid bias (blinding and randomisation techniques).

The investigator and the monitor are responsible for ensuring that the data collected are of a high quality. The statistician must ensure the integrity of the data during their processing and, in addition, that an account is made of missing, unused or spurious data during the statistical analysis. These omissions must be documented to enable a suitable review of the results.

The results of the statistical analyses and findings are presented in the Final Report). The statistician must also ensure that the results of the statistical analyses are presented in a manner which helps the interpretation of the clinical importance of changes.

Quality assurance

The sponsor is responsible for ensuring that all the procedures involved in conducting studies to GCP are subjected to quality assurance checks. Many companies have set up quality assurance (QA) groups to check that each stage of the clinical trial is performed correctly and that data are reliable and that they have been processed properly. In addition, the QA department will check that the company is in compliance with its own SOPs. Obviously, the QA personnel must be independent of the clinical research department.

Audits of trials may be conducted by the company's QA department at any time and this should be a regular and ongoing process. When audits are undertaken by regulatory authorities they are called inspections; here, representatives of the authority visit the company and inspect trial files and documents to determine the reliability and validity of data that will be submitted as part of a product licence application. Obviously if SOPs and GCP have not been followed it is possible that data may not be accepted.

The Trial Master File

Probably the most important role for monitors, secretaries and administrators in clinical research departments is the maintenance of the Trial Master File. Study files should be kept up-to-date at all times, not only as an aid to the monitor whose heavy workload can be handled more effectively if the trial files are regularly updated, but also in the event of audits and inspections. The company must be able to demonstrate that it has fulfilled the requirements of GCP and the only way to do this is to document every action during a trial.

A full listing of the essential documents regarded as the minimum required can be found in the appendix to the ICH GCP Guidelines (Appended). The book "Which Documents, Why?" (see *Further Reading*, page 61) describes the investigator's documentation requirements.

Problems of implementing GCP

The extra administrative workloads caused by GCP have been burdensome on monitors, secretaries and administrators. The monitor is no longer able to manage as many studies as they did prior to the implementation of GCP – monitoring visits now take much longer and the amount of work which has to be undertaken at each study site has increased. This in turn has led to greater staffing requirements in companies or a reduction in the size of its clinical research programme. Furthermore the costs of clinical research has increased reflecting these greater staff costs and increased fees to investigators who have also had an increase in their workload when taking part in a trial.

One major issue in implementing GCP has been a change in attitude towards the confidentiality of patient records. GCP makes it necessary for monitors to check the data recorded by investigators in CRFs against notes made in confidential patient files held by the doctor. This is called source data verification (SDV). Whilst most investigators now allow monitors to directly compare CRF entries with the patient files, providing the monitor behaves in a responsible and professional way towards confidentiality of information seen, some still will not allow this process to take place. These investigators are no longer acceptable if the study is to be performed in accordance with ICH GCP.

As GCP becomes more understood by investigators and companies alike the initial problems of implementing a more administrative and bureaucratic system will diminish and the real benefits of adhering to these strict guidelines will become more obvious.

Conclusion

GCP should always be implemented in clinical trials and all companies have addressed this requirement by writing their own SOPs which should be adhered to at all times. In the early stages of implementation, companies should test the practicability of their SOPs and, if necessary, make changes to ensure that they may be more readily followed. SOPs must be frequently reviewed to ensure that they meet any changes in GCP Guidelines which may occur from time to time by the issue of new directives.

All staff involved in clinical trials have a responsibility to ensure that SOPs are followed; a great role is played by the non-technical personnel who often document and administer each study. Additional strain is placed on trial monitors and investigators alike to conform to the often burdensome bureaucracy associated with GCP and a more than cursory knowledge of trial methodology and good clinical practice will make a secretary or trial administrator an invaluable member of the clinical research team.

*Clinical research management is not for the faint-hearted –
enthusiasm, a keen eye for detail, good organisational skills, the
ability to motivate, be diplomatic, add up and work effectively under
extreme pressures are essential qualities for the trial organiser.*

4

Further reading

The following publications may be read or used as reference texts to supplement the contents of this book.

Basic texts

Boylander A, Bolander D O.
The New Webster's Medical Dictionary.
The Lewtan Line, Hartford, Connecticut, USA, 1992 (ASI 67230).

Winslade J, Hutchinson D R.
Dictionary of Clinical Research.
Brookwood Medical Publications, UK, 1992 (ISBN 1-874409-00-5).

Hutchinson D R.
Critical path analysis of the clinical trial: improving efficiency and cost effectiveness.
American Journal of Clinical Research 1992; **1**: 3 – 14.

Hutchinson D R.
A causality algorithm to determine the relationship of adverse events to drug therapy.
British Journal of Clinical Research 1991; **2**: 157 – 163.

Hutchinson DR.
The Trial Investigator's GCP Handbook.
Brookwood Medical Publications, UK, 1997 (ISBN 1-874409-76-5).

Hutchinson D R.
Which Documents, Why?
Brookwood Medical Publications, UK, 1997 (ISBN 1-874409-81-1).

ICH Harmonised Tripartite Guideline for Good Clinical Practice
Brookwood Medical Publications, UK, 1996 (ISBN 1-874409-71-4).

Advanced reading

Lock S, Wells F (eds).
Fraud and misconduct in Medical Research. Publ. BMJ Publishing
Group, London, 1993 (ISBN 0-7279-0757-3).

Spilker B.
Guide to clinical trials. Raven Press, New York, 1991.
(ISBN 0-88167-767-1).

Spilker B.
Data collection forms in clinical trials. Raven Press, New York, 1991.
(ISBN 0-88167-759-0).

Spilker B, Cramer J A.
Patient recruitment in clinical trials. Raven Press, New York
(ISBN 0-88167-931-3).

Appendix 1: The Declaration Of Helsinki

*Recommendations guiding physicians in biomedical
research involving human subjects*

Adopted by the 18th World Medical Assembly, Helsinki, Finland June 1964,
and amended by the 29th World Medical Assembly, Tokyo, Japan October 1975,
35th World Medical Assembly, Venice, Italy, October 1983,
41st World Medical Assembly, Hong Kong, September 1989
and the 48th General Assembly, Somerset West,
Republic of South Africa, October 1996.

Introduction

It is the mission of the physician to safeguard the health of the people. His or her
knowledge and conscience are dedicated to the fulfilment of this mission.

The Declaration of Geneva of the World Medical Association binds the physician
with the words: "The health of my patient will be my first considerations." And the
International Code of Medical Ethics declares that "A physician shall act only in the
patient's interest when providing medical care which might have the effect of
weakening the physical and mental condition of the patient".

The purpose of biomedical research involving human subjects must be to improve
diagnostic, therapeutic and prophylactic procedures and the understanding of the
aetiology and pathogenesis of disease.

In current medical practice most diagnostic, therapeutic or prophylactic procedure
involve hazards. This applies especially to biomedical research.

Medical progress is based on research which ultimately must rest in part on
experimentation involving human subjects.

In the field of biomedical research a fundamental distinction must be recognised
between medical research in which the aim is essentially diagnostic or therapeutic
for a patient and medical research the essential object of which is purely scientific
and without direct diagnostic or therapeutic value to the person subjected to the
research.

Special caution must be exercised in the conduct of research which may affect the
environment and the welfare of animals used for research must be respected.

Because it is essential that the results of laboratory experiments be applied to human beings to further scientific knowledge and to help suffering humanity, the World Medical Association has prepared the following recommendations as a guide to every physician in biomedical research involving human subjects. They should be kept under review in the future. It must be stressed that the standards as drafted are only a guide to physicians all over the world. Physicians are not relieved from criminal, civil and ethical responsibilities under the laws of their own countries.

1. Basic Principles

1 Biomedical research involving human subjects must conform to generally accepted scientific principles and should be based an adequately performed laboratory and animal experimentation and on a thorough knowledge of the scientific literature.

2 The design and performance of each experimental procedure involving human subjects should be clearly formulated in an experimental protocol which should be transmitted for consideration, comment and guidance to a specially appointed committee independent of the investigator and the sponsor provided that this independent committee is in conformity with the laws and regulations of the country in which the research experiment is performed.

3 Biomedical research involving human subjects should be conducted only by scientifically qualified persons and under the supervision of a clinically competent medical person. The responsibility for the human subject must always rest with a medically qualified person and never rest on the subject of the research, even though the subject has given his or her consent.

4 Biomedical research involving human subjects cannot legitimately be carried out unless the importance of the objective is in proportion to the inherent risk to the subject.

5 Every biomedical research project involving human subjects should be preceded by careful assessment of predictable risks in comparison with foreseeable benefits to the subject or to others. Concern for the interests of the subject must always prevail over the interest of science and society.

6 The right of the research subject to safeguard his or her integrity must always be respected. Every precaution should be taken to respect the privacy of the subject and to minimise the impact of the study on the subject's physical and mental integrity and on the personality of the subject.

7 Physicians should abstain from engaging in research projects involving human subjects unless they are satisfied that the hazards involved are believed to be predictable. Physicians should cease any investigation if the hazards are found to outweigh the potential benefits.

8 In publications of the results of his or her research, the physician is obliged to preserve the accuracy of the results. Reports of experimentation not in accordance with the principles laid down in this Declaration should not be accepted for publication.

9 In any research on human beings, each potential subject must be adequately informed of the aims, methods, anticipated benefits and potential hazards of the study, and the discomfort it may entail. He or she should be informed that he or she is at liberty to abstain from participating in the study and that he or she is free to withdraw his or her consent to participation at any time. The physician should then obtain the subject's freely-given informed consent, preferably in writing.

10 When obtaining informed consent for the research project the physician should be particularly cautious if the subject is in a dependent relationship to him or her or may consent under duress. In that case the informed consent should be obtained by a physician who is not engaged in the investigation and who is completely independent of this official relationship.

11 In case of legal incompetence, informed consent should be obtained from the legal guardian in accordance with national legislation. Where physical or mental incapacity makes it impossible to obtain informed consent, or when the subject is a minor, permission from the responsible relative replaces that of the subject in accordance with national legislation.

   Whenever the minor child is in fact able to give consent, the minor's consent must be obtained in addition to the consent of the minor's legal guardian.

12 The research protocol should always contain a statement of the ethical considerations involved and should indicate that the principles enunciated in the present Declaration are complied with:

II Medical Research Combined With Professional Care (Clinical Research)

1 In the treatment of the sick person, the physician must be free to use a new diagnostic and therapeutic measure, if in his or her judgement it offers hope of saving life, re-establishing health or alleviating suffering.

2   The potential benefits, hazards and discomfort of the new method should be weighed against the advantages of the best current diagnostic and therapeutic methods.

3   In any medical study, every patient – including those of a control group, if any – should be assured of the best proven diagnostic and therapeutic method. This does not exclude the use of inert placebo in studies where no proven diagnostic or therapeutic method exists.

4   The refusal of the patient to participate in a study must never interfere with the physician-patient relationship.

5   If the physician considers it essential not to obtain informed consent, the specific reasons for this proposal should be stated in the experimental protocol for transmission to the independent committee (1,2).

6   The physician can combine medical research with professional care, the objective being acquisition of new medical knowledge, only to the extent that medical research is justified by its potential diagnostic or therapeutic value for the patient.

III Non-Therapeutic Biomedical Research Involving
Human Subjects (Non-clinical biomedical research)

1   In the purely scientific application of medical research carried out on a human being, it is the duty of the physician to remain the protector of the life and health of that person on whom biomedical research is being carried out.

2   The subjects should be volunteers - either healthy persons or patients for whom the experimental design is not related to the patient's illness.

3   The investigator or investigating team should discontinue the research if in his/her or their judgement it may, if continued, be harmful to the individual.

4   In research on man, the interest of science and society should never take precedence over considerations related to the well-being of the subject.

Appendix 2: Essential Documents For The Conduct Of A Clinical Trial

8.1 Introduction

Essential Documents are those documents which individually and collectively permit evaluation of the conduct of a trial and the quality of the data produced. These documents serve to demonstrate the compliance of the investigator, sponsor and monitor with the standards of Good Clinical Practice and with all applicable regulatory requirements.

Essential Documents also serve a number of other important purposes. Filing essential documents at the investigator/ institution and sponsor sites in a timely manner can greatly assist in the successful management of a trial by the investigator, sponsor and monitor. These documents are also the ones which are usually audited by the sponsor's independent audit function and inspected by the regulatory authority (ies) as part of the process to confirm the validity of the trial conduct and the integrity of data collected.

The minimum list of essential documents which has been developed follows. The various documents are grouped in three sections according to the stage of the trial during which they will normally be generated: 1) before the clinical phase of the trial commences, 2) during the clinical conduct of the trial, and 3) after completion or termination of the trial. A description is given of the purpose of each document, and whether it should be filed in either the investigator/institution or sponsor files, or both. It is acceptable to combine some of the documents, provided the individual elements are readily identifiable.

Trial master files should be established at the beginning of the trial, both at the investigator/institution's site and at the sponsor's office. A final close-out of a trial can only be done when the monitor has reviewed both investigator/institution and sponsor files and confirmed that all necessary documents are in the appropriate files.

Any or all of the documents addressed in this guideline may be subject to, and should be available for, audit by the sponsor's auditor and inspection by the regulatory authority(ies).

Title of document	Purpose	Located in Files of	
		Investigator/ Institution	Sponsor

8.2 Before the Clinical Phase of the Trial Commences

During this planning stage the following documents should be generated and should be on file before the trial formally starts

Title of document	Purpose	Investigator/ Institution	Sponsor
8.2.1 INVESTIGATOR'S BROCHURE	To document that relevant and current scientific information about the investigational product has been provided to the investigator	X	X
8.2.2 SIGNED PROTOCOL AND AMENDMENTS, IF ANY, AND SAMPLE CASE REPORT FORM (CRF)	To document investigator and sponsor agreement to the protocol/ amendment(s) and CRF	X	X
8.2.3 INFORMATION GIVEN TO TRIAL SUBJECT – INFORMED CONSENT FORM (including all applicable translations)	To document the informed consent	X	X
– ANY OTHER WRITTEN INFORMATION	To document that subjects will be given appropriate written information (content and wording) to support their ability to give fully informed consent	X	X
– ADVERTISEMENT FOR SUBJECT RECRUITMENT (if used)	To document that recruitment measures are appropriate and not coercive	X	
8.2.4 FINANCIAL ASPECTS OF THE TRIAL	To document the financial agreement between the investigator/institution and the sponsor for the trial	X	X
8.2.5 INSURANCE STATEMENT (where required)	To document that compensation to subject(s) for trial-related injury will be available	X	X

Title of document	Purpose	Located in Files of	
		Investigator/ Institution	**Sponsor**
8.2.6 SIGNED AGREEMENT BETWEEN INVOLVED PARTIES, e.g.:	To document agreements		
– investigator/institution and sponsor		X	X
– investigator/institution and CRO		X	X (where required)
– sponsor and CRO		X	X
– investigator/institution and authority(ies) (where required)			X
8.2.7 DATED, DOCUMENTED APPROVAL/ FAVOURABLE OPINION OF INSTITUTIONAL REVIEW BOARD (IRB)/INDEPENDENT ETHICS COMMITTEE (IEC) OF THE FOLLOWING: – protocol and any amendments – CRF (if applicable) – informed consent form(s) – any other written information to be provided to the subject(s) – advertisement for subject recruitment (if used) – subject compensation (if any) – any other documents given approval/ favourable opinion	To document that the trial has been subject to IRB/IEC review and given approval/favourable opinion. To identify the version number and date of the document(s)	X	X
8.2.8 INSTITUTIONAL REVIEW BOARD/ INDEPENDENT ETHICS COMMITTEE COMPOSITION	To document that the IRB/IEC is constituted in agreement with GCP	X	X (where required)
8.2.9 REGULATORY AUTHORITY(IES) AUTHORISATION/ APPROVAL/ NOTIFICATION OF PROTOCOL (where required)	To document appropriate authorisation/approval/ notification by the regulatory authority(ies) has been obtained prior to initiation of the trial in compliance with the applicable regulatory requirement(s)	X (where required)	X (where required)

Title of document	Purpose	Located in Files of	
		Investigator/ Institution	Sponsor
8.2.10 CURRICULUM VITAE AND/OR OTHER REL-EVANT DOCUMENTS EVIDENCING QUAL-IFICATIONS OF INVES-TIGATOR(S) AND SUB-INVESTIGATOR(S)	To document qualifications and eligibility to conduct trial and/or provide medical supervision of subjects	X	X
8.2.11 NORMAL VALUE(S) /RANGE(S) FOR MEDICAL/ LABORATORY/ TECHNICAL PRO-CEDURE(S) AND/OR TEST(S) INCLUDED IN THE PROTOCOL	To document normal values and/or ranges of the tests	X	X
8.2.12 MEDICAL/ LABORATORY/TECH-NICAL PROCEDURES/ TESTS – certification or – accreditation or – established quality control and/or external quality assessment or – other validation (where required)	To document competence of facility to perform required test(s), and support reliability of results	X (where required)	X
8.2.13 SAMPLE OF LABEL(S) ATTACHED TO INVESTIGATIONAL PRODUCT CONTAINER(S)	To document compliance with applicable labelling regulations and appropriateness of instructions provided to the subjects		X
8.2.14 INSTRUCTIONS FOR HANDLING OF INVESTIGATIONAL PRODUCT(S) AND TRIAL-RELATED MATERIALS (if not included in protocol or Investigator's Brochure)	To document instructions needed to ensure proper storage, packaging, dispensing and disposition of investigational products and trial-related materials	X	X
8.2.15 SHIPPING RECORDS FOR INVESTIGATIONAL PRODUCT(S) AND TRIAL-RELATED MATERIALS	To document shipment dates, batch numbers and method of shipment of investigational product(s) and trial-related materials. Allows tracking of product batch, review of shipping conditions, and accountability	X	X

Title of document	Purpose	Located in Files of	
		Investigator/ Institution	**Sponsor**
8.2.16 CERTIFICATE(S) OF ANALYSIS OF INVESTIGATIONAL PRODUCT(S) SHIPPED	To document identity, purity, and strength of investigational product(s) to be used in the trial		X
8.2.17 DECODING PROCEDURES FOR BLINDED TRIALS	To document how, in case of an emergency, identity of blinded investigational product can be revealed without breaking the blind for the remaining subjects' treatment	X	X (third party if applicable)
8.2.18 MASTER RANDOMISATION LIST	To document method for randomisation of trial population		X (third party if applicable)
8.2.19 PRE-TRIAL MONITORING REPORT	To document that the site is suitable for the trial (may be combined with 8.2.20)		X
8.2.20 TRIAL INITIATION MONITORING REPORT	To document that trial procedures were reviewed with the investigator and the investigator's trial staff (may be combined with 8.2.19)	X	X

8.3 During the Clinical Conduct of the Trial

In addition to having on file the above documents, the following should be added to the files during the trial as evidence that all new relevant information is documented as it becomes available

8.3.1 INVESTIGATOR'S BROCHURE UPDATES	To document that investigator is informed in a timely manner of relevant information as it becomes available	X	X
8.3.2 ANY REVISION TO: – protocol/amendment(s) and CRF – informed consent form – any other written information provided to subjects – advertisement for subject recruitment(if used)	To document revisions of these trial related documents that take effect during trial	X	X

Title of document	Purpose	Located in Files of	
		Investigator/ Institution	Sponsor

8.3.3 DATED, DOCUMENTED APPROVAL/ FAVOUR-ABLE OPINION OF INSTITUTIONAL REVIEW BOARD (IRB) /INDEPENDENT ETHICS COMMITTEE (IEC) OF THE FOLLOWING:
– protocol amendment(s)
– revision(s) of:
  – informed consent form
  – any other written information to be provided to the subject
  – advertisement for subject recruitment (if used)
– any other documents given approval/favourable opinion
– continuing review of trial (where required)
	To document that the amendment(s) and/or revision(s) have been subject to IRB/IEC review and were given approval/favourable opinion. To identify the version number and date of the document(s).	X	X

8.3.4 REGULATORY AUTHORITY(IES) AUTHORISATIONS/ APPROVALS/ NOTIFICATIONS WHERE REQUIRED FOR: – protocol amendment(s) and other documents	To document compliance with applicable regulatory requirements	X (where required)	X
8.3.5 CURRICULUM VITAE FOR NEW INVESTIGA-TOR(S) AND/OR SUB-INVESTIGATOR(S)	(see 8.2.10)	X	X
8.3.6 UPDATES TO NORMAL VALUE(S)/RANGE(S) FOR MEDICAL/ LABORATORY/ TECH-NICAL PROCEDURE(S)/ TEST(S) INCLUDED IN THE PROTOCOL	To document normal values and ranges that are revised during the trial (see 8.2.11)	X	X

Title of document	Purpose	Located in Files of Investigator/ Institution	Sponsor
8.3.7 UPDATES OF MEDICAL/ LABORATORY/TECH-NICAL PROCEDURES/ TESTS – certification or – accreditation or – established quality control and/or external quality assessment or – other validation (where required)	To document that tests remain adequate throughout the trial period (see 8.2.12)	X (where required)	X
8.3.8 DOCUMENTATION OF INVESTIGATIONAL PRODUCT(S) AND TRIAL-RELATED MATERIALS SHIPMENT	(see 8.2.15)	X	X
8.3.9 CERTIFICATE(S) OF ANALYSIS FOR NEW BATCHES OF INVESTIGATIONAL PRODUCTS	(see 8.2.16)		X
8.3.10 MONITORING VISIT REPORTS	To document site visits by, and findings of, the monitor		X
8.3.11 RELEVANT COMMUNICATIONS OTHER THAN SITE VISITS – letters – meeting notes – notes of telephone calls	To document any agreements or significant discussions regarding trial administration, protocol violations, trial conduct, adverse event (AE) reporting	X	X
8.3.12 SIGNED INFORMED CONSENT FORMS	To document that consent is obtained in accordance with GCP and protocol and dated prior to participation of each subject in trial. Also to document direct access permission (see 8.2.3)	X	
8.3.13 SOURCE DOCUMENTS	To document the existence of the subject and substantiate integrity of trial data collected. To include original documents related to the trial, to medical treatment, and history of subject	X	

Title of document	Purpose	Located in Files of	
		Investigator/ Institution	**Sponsor**
8.3.14 SIGNED, DATED AND COMPLETED CASE REPORT FORMS (CRF)	To document that the investigator or authorised member of the investigator's staff confirms the observations recorded	X (copy)	X (original)
8.3.15 DOCUMENTATION OF CRF CORRECTIONS	To document all changes/additions or corrections made to CRF after initial data were recorded	X (copy)	X (original)
8.3.16 NOTIFICATION BY ORIGINATING INVESTIGATOR TO SPONSOR OF SERIOUS ADVERSE EVENTS AND RELATED REPORTS	Notification by originating investigator to sponsor of serious adverse events and related reports in accordance with 4.11	X	X
8.3.17 NOTIFICATION BY SPONSOR AND/OR INVESTIGATOR, WHERE APPLICABLE, TO REGULATORY AUTHORITY(IES) AND IRB(S)/IEC(S) OF UNEXPECTED SERIOUS ADVERSE DRUG REACTIONS AND OF OTHER SAFETY INFORMATION	Notification by sponsor and/or investigator, where applicable, to regulatory authorities and IRB(s)/ IEC(s) of unexpected serious adverse drug reactions in accordance with 5.17 and 4.11.1 and of other safety information in accordance with 5.16.2	X (where required)	X
8.3.18 NOTIFICATION BY SPONSOR TO INVESTIGATORS OF SAFETY INFORMATION	Notification by sponsor to investigators of safety information in accordance with 5.16.2	X	X
8.3.19 INTERIM OR ANNUAL REPORTS TO IRB/IEC AND AUTHORITY(IES)	Interim or annual reports provided to IRB/IEC in accordance with 4.10 and to authority(ies) in accordance with 5.17.3	X	X (where required)
8.3.20 SUBJECT SCREENING LOG	To document identification of subjects who entered pre-trial screening	X	X (where required)

Title of document	Purpose	Located in Files of	
		Investigator/ Institution	Sponsor
8.3.21 SUBJECT IDENTIFICATION CODE LIST	To document that investigator/ institution keeps a confidential list of names of all subjects allocated to trial numbers on enrolling in the trial. Allows investigator/institution to reveal identity of any subject	X	
8.3.22 SUBJECT ENROLMENT LOG	To document chronological enrolment of subjects by trial number	X	
8.3.23 INVESTIGATIONAL PRODUCTS ACCOUNT- ABILITY AT THE SITE	To document that investigational product(s) have been used according to the protocol	X	X
8.3.24 SIGNATURE SHEET	To document signatures and initials of all persons authorised to make entries and/or corrections on CRFs	X	X
8.3.25 RECORD OF RETAINED BODY FLUIDS/TISSUE SAMPLES (IF ANY)	To document location and identification of retained samples if assays need to be repeated	X	X

8.4 After completion or termination of the trial

After completion or termination of the trial, all of the documents identified in sections 8.2 and 8.3 should be in the file together with the following

8.4.1 INVESTIGATIONAL PRODUCT(S) ACCOUNT- ABILITY AT SITE	To document that the investigational product(s) have been used according to the protocol. To documents the final accounting of investigational product(s) received at the site, dispensed to subjects, returned by the subjects, and returned to sponsor	X	X
8.4.2 DOCUMENTATION OF INVESTIGATIONAL PRODUCT DESTRUCTION	To document destruction of unused investigational products by sponsor or at site	X (if destroyed at site)	X

Title of document	Purpose	Located in Files of	
		Investigator/ Institution	Sponsor
8.4.3 COMPLETED SUBJECT IDENTIFICATION CODE LIST	To permit identification of all subjects enrolled in the trial in case follow-up is required. List should be kept in a confidential manner and for agreed upon time	X	
8.4.4 AUDIT CERTIFICATE (if available)	To document that audit was performed		X
8.4.5 FINAL TRIAL CLOSE-OUT MONITORING REPORT	To document that all activities required for trial close-out are completed, and copies of essential documents are held in the appropriate files		X
8.4.6 TREATMENT ALLOCATION AND DECODING DOCUMENTATION	Returned to sponsor to document any decoding that may have occurred		X
8.4.7 FINAL REPORT BY INVESTIGATOR TO IRB/IEC WHERE REQUIRED, AND WHERE APPLICABLE, TO THE REGULATORY AUTHORITY(IES)	To document completion of the trial	X	
8.4.8 CLINICAL STUDY REPORT	To document results and interpretation of trial	X (if applicable)	X

Index

A a
administrator 50
adverse drug reaction (ADR) 29
adverse events (AEs) 29 – 31
animal tests 2 – 3
archiving 56
audits 57

B b
blinding 20
briefing, pre-study 39

C c
case record forms (CRFs) 11 – 13, 36
  adverse events 30, 31
  data recording 55
  data verification 43, 54, 58
Clinical Trial Exemption (CTX) 9
clinical trials 5, 8 – 25
  allocating treatment 18 – 19
  balancing treatment groups 20 – 21
  blinding 20
  controls 14 – 15
  cost effectiveness 7 – 8
  critical path 32 – 45
  design 15 – 17
  measuring efficacy 26 – 28
  measuring safety 28 – 31
  monitoring 42 – 43, 58
  multicentre 17 – 18, 21, 35, 39
  objectives 13
  protocol 10 – 11, 35 – 36
  records, *see* case record forms

regulatory aspects 9 – 10, 36 – 38
stages 34 – 45
subjects, *see* healthy volunteers; patients
termination 43
variability and 21 – 22
compensation 9, 51 – 53
computer records 55
confidentiality 43, 58
consent 9, 51 – 52
controls 14 – 15
"correspondence test" 38
cost effectiveness, clinical trials 7 – 8
CRFs, *see* case record forms
crossover studies 15 – 17
curriculum vitae 38

D d
data
  archiving 56
  entry 43
  recording 55 – 56
  statistical analysis 49, 56 – 57
  verification, source (SDV) 43, 54 – 55, 59
Declaration of Helsinki 9, 51
Department of Health 6, 9 – 10
design, trial 15 – 17
dose
  choosing 15
  optimum 4
double blind studies 20, 24
double dummy technique 24, 25

drug development 1 – 8
  application for product
  licence 5 – 6
  difficult decisions 5
  health economics 7
  initial tests 2 – 3
  need for cost effective
  research 7 – 8
  Phase I studies 3
  Phase II studies 3 – 4
  Phase III studies 5
  post-marketing (Phase IV)
  studies 6 – 7
  risk-benefit ratio 4
drug discovery 2

E e
economics, health 7
elderly patients 5
Ethics Committee 9, 36 – 38, 51 –
52
European Community, GCP
guidelines 37, 47, 49 – 56

F f
Final Report 44 – 45
Food and Drug Administration
(FDA) 9, 46
fraud 47

G g
GCP, *see* Good Clinical Practice
generic drugs 2, 8
Good Clinical Practice (GCP)
46 – 60
  European Community guidelines
  37, 47, 49 – 57

  problems of implementing
  58 – 59
  rationale 46 – 47
  responsibilities 50
  Standard Operating Procedures
  and 50
Good Clinical Research Practice
(GCRP), *see* Good Clinical
Practice

H h
Hamilton Depression Rating Scale
26
Hawthorne effect 23 – 24
health economics 7
healthy volunteers 3 – 4, 25

I i
indemnity insurance 51
information 51
inspections 57
institutional review board (IRB)
37 – 38
investigators 36, 38-39
  data handling 55, 56
  Ethics Committee approval 51
  payments 25
  responsibilities 54 – 55
  selection 32, 38 – 39
  study protocol and 35

J j
journals, medical 45

L l
licensed-in drugs 2

M m

matched pairs 17
materials, study 39 – 40
Medicines Control Agency (MCA)
6, 9
monitoring 42 – 43, 58
monitors, trial
   data verification 43, 54
   responsibilities 53 – 54
   site assessment 39
multicentre studies 17 – 18, 21,
35, 39

O o

open studies 20

P p

paper, self-duplicating (NCR)
11 – 12
parallel group design 17, 18
patients
   confidentiality 46, 58
   Phase II studies 4
   protection 8 – 9, 51 – 52
   recruitment 40 – 42
   variability 21 – 22
payments 24 – 25
pharmaceutical companies
   drug development 1 – 8
   Standard Operating Procedures
   (SOPs) 10, 42, 50, 59
   see also sponsors
pharmacist 38 – 40
Phase I studies 3, 10
Phase II studies 3 – 4
Phase III studies 5
Phase IV (post-marketing) studies
6 – 7

placebo 14 – 16, 22 – 24
   double blind studies 24
   response 22 – 24, 28
planning 34 – 35
post-marketing studies (Phase IV)
6 – 7
Post-Marketing Surveillance 6
pre-study briefing 39
Product Licence (PL) 5 – 6, 7
protocol, clinical trial 10 – 11,
35 – 36
publication of results 45

Q q

quality assurance (QA) 44,
57 – 58
questionnaires 26

R r

randomisation 18 – 19, 20 – 21
   stratified 21
rating scales 26 – 27
records
   confidentiality 45, 58 – 59
   study, *see* case record forms
recruitment, patient 40 – 42
regulatory authorities 36 – 38, 45
   approval of trials 9 – 10
   inspections 57
responsibilities 50 – 55
risk-benefit ratio 4
"run-in" phase 15, 16, 18

S s

safety, measuring 28 – 31
secretary 50, 59
self-duplicating (NCR) paper
11 – 12

single blind studies 20
site assessment 39
SOPs, *see* Standard Operating
Procedures
source data verification (SDV) 43,
54 – 55, 59
sponsors
    data handling 55
    quality assurance 57 – 58
    responsibilities 52 – 53
    see also pharmaceutical
    companies
Standard Operating Procedures
(SOPs) 10, 42, 50 – 51, 58
statistical analysis 43 – 44, 57
statistician 43 – 44, 56 – 57
sub-groups 21

T t
termination, study 43
Trial Master File 58
twins, identical 17

V v
 variability 21 – 22
visual analogue scale (VAS) 27

W w
"wash-out" period 15 – 16